MCQs in Otolaryngology

MCQs in Otolaryngology

Second Edition

James W. Fairley BSc FRCS MS
Consultant ENT Surgeon
William Harvey Hospital
Ashford, Kent

R. S. Dhillon FRCS
Consultant ENT Surgeon
Northwick Park Hospital
Harrow, Middlesex

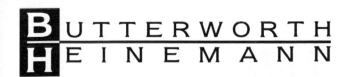

OXFORD   AUCKLAND   BOSTON   JOHANNESBURG   MELBOURNE   NEW DELHI

Butterworth-Heinemann
Linacre House, Jordan Hill, Oxford OX2 8DP
225 Wildwood Avenue, Woburn, MA 01801-2041
A division of Reed Educational and Professional Publishing Ltd

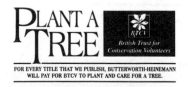 A member of the Reed Elsevier plc group

First published by the Macmillan Press Ltd 1989
Second edition 1999

© James Fairley and R S Dhillon 1999

British Library Cataloguing in Publication Data
A catalogue record for this book is available from the British Library

Library of Congress Cataloguing in Publication Data
A catalogue record for this book is available from the Library of Congress

ISBN 0 7506 2165 6

Printed and bound in Great Britain by Biddles Ltd, Guildford and King's Lynn

PLANT A TREE

British Trust for Conservation Volunteers

FOR EVERY TITLE THAT WE PUBLISH, BUTTERWORTH-HEINEMANN
WILL PAY FOR BTCV TO PLANT AND CARE FOR A TREE.

Contents

Preface to the first edition

Like them or loathe them, multiple-choice questions are firmly established in undergraduate and postgraduate medical education. Their importance can only increase as computers are used more and more to automate the assessment of students.

This book is designed primarily as a revision aid. It is particularly suitable for DLO and FRCS candidates throughout the world, but it could be used with profit by undergraduates. It can be used to discover gaps in knowledge and to reinforce what has been learned from standard textbooks. We have included short notes with the answers. These provide further information and try to explain why we favour a given response in cases where there may be disagreement.

There are 1590 questions here, arranged as 318 stems, each with 5 independent true/false statements. All major areas of otolaryngology are covered. The questions are ordered by subject in 5 sections: ear; nose and sinuses; larynx and tracheobronchial tree; mouth, pharynx and oesophagus; and general and related topics.

The subject matter is covered in the standard British ENT textbooks. We have made extensive use of Scott-Brown, both fourth and fifth editions, the ear, nose and throat volumes of Rob and Smith's *Operative Surgery*, Groves and Gray's *Synopsis of Otolaryngology*, Stell and Maran's *Head and Neck Surgery*, and Mawson and Ludman's *Diseases of the Ear*.

When compiling MCQs it is tempting to stick to factual or uncontroversial issues. This artificial restriction takes a lot of the interest out of the subject. We have included controversial aspects of clinical practice, as well as basic anatomy, physiology and pathology. We recognize that the reduction of complex issues to a series of true/false statements can never be perfect. No doubt some experienced colleagues will disagree with our answers. Perhaps they will take consolation from the fact that in real life the unfortunate candidate not only has to know what is right, but also to know what the examiner knows is right!

We are grateful to the Director and staff of the Ferens Institute of Otolaryngology, under whose auspices the book was produced. We also thank our colleagues and students at the Royal Ear Hospital, the Middlesex Hospital and Mount Vernon Hospital for their helpful suggestions. In particular we would like to thank Mr Richard Williams, Mr Graham Fraser, Mr Garry Glover and Mr Phillip Robinson for their careful reading of the questions. They have all pointed out ambiguities and inconsistencies which bedevil the MCQ compiler. Any faults which remain are the authors' responsibility. Finally, we would like to thank our wives, Georgina and Sylvia, for their continued support during the two-year gestation period of the book.

R.S.D.
J.W.F.
London, 1989

Preface to the second edition

In the ten years since our first edition of multiple choice questions in otolaryngology, much has changed but much has remained the same. Anatomy does not alter, as Professor Slome used to remind Primary FRCS candidates in London. Therefore most of our anatomy questions and answers remain the same. Along with the rest of the book, they are now cross-referenced into Scott-Brown's *Otolaryngology*, 6th edition (1997), Oxford: Butterworth-Heinemann, ISBN 0 7506 1935 X and Gray and Hawthorne's *Synopsis of Otolaryngology*, 5th edition (1992), Oxford: Butterworth-Heinemann, ISBN 0 7506 1358 0. This MCQ book is best used with the established texts, to probe your knowledge and to stimulate further reading. Slome taught physiology, and he quipped that for MCQs you can ask the same questions over the years, but just change the answers. In clinical practice, however, the questions themselves have to change. This we have done, to keep pace with new developments such as FESS, MRI scanning, AIDS and other developing areas. It remains true that reduction of complex issues to a series of true/false statements can never be perfect. Any imperfections that remain, despite the careful attention of Butterworth-Heinemann's proof readers, are, of course, entirely the fault of the authors.

James W. Fairley
Ashford, Kent

The ear

1. **In foetal development:**
   a. There are six visceral arches and five visceral clefts.
   b. The facial nerve supplies the second or hyoid arch.
   c. The pharyngeal pouches are formed from the ectodermal furrows.
   d. The tuberculum impar, the lingual swellings and the hypobranchial eminence form the tongue.
   e. In the adult, the sulcus terminalis in the tongue marks the site of the thyroid rudiment.

2. **Development of the foetal ear:**
   a. The Eustachian tube is formed from the ectoderm of the first visceral cleft.
   b. The auricle develops from the first visceral cleft as a series of six tubercles.
   c. The stapes footplate is derived from ectoderm.
   d. The inner ear is developed from ectoderm, and has reached full adult size by the fourth foetal month.
   e. The stapes superstructure, styloid process and hyoid are derived from the first visceral arch.

1. *Synopsis 3–4, 287*
    a. False There are six of each.
    b. True   Each visceral arch has its own nerve supply. The
              mandibular division of the trigeminal nerve supplies
              the mandibular arch (first); the facial, the hyoid arch
              (second); the glossopharyngeal (third), the vagus and
              accessory the remainder.
    c. False They are formed from the endodermal furrows.
    d. True.
    e. False The site is the foramen caecum.

2. *Synopsis 4–6; Scott-Brown 1/1/6–11*
    a. False It is formed from the endoderm of the tubotympanic
              recess. The ectoderm of the first cleft forms the
              external auditory canal.
    b. True   These eventually fuse to form the definitive pinna.
    c. False The stapes head, neck and crura are derived from
              mesoderm of the second visceral arch, and the
              footplate from the otic capsule. Hence otosclerosis,
              a disease of the otic capsule, primarily affects the
              footplate region.
    d. True.
    e. False The bone and cartilaginous derivatives are: first
              arch – malleus, incus, Meckel's cartilage; second
              arch – stapes superstructure, styloid process, stylohyoid
              ligament, hyoid body; third arch – hyoid inferior body
              and greater cornu; fourth arch – thyroid and epiglottis;
              sixth arch – arytenoids.

3. **Development of the temporal bone:**
   a. The tympanic ring and squama are ossified in cartilage.
   b. The foramen of Huschke is a defect in the tympanic ring.
   c. Ossification of the endosteal layer of the petromastoid may be defective, particularly in the vicinity of the fissula ante-fenestram.
   d. The facial nerve is well protected at birth by the mastoid process.
   e. In the infant, the mastoid antrum lies below the tympanic cavity and about 5 mm deep to the bony surface.

4. **Development of the mastoid process:**
   a. The diploic type has large and numerous air cells containing marrow spaces.
   b. Wittmack suggested that disease processes, in particular infantile otitis media, prevent normal mastoid pneumatization by interfering with normal absorption of diploë.
   c. Diamant suggested that hypocellularity of the mastoid is merely a normal variant.
   d. Both the Tumarkin and the mastoid plate distraction theories of mastoid pneumatization depend on satisfactory middle ear ventilation.
   e. Only about 50 per cent of mastoids are pneumatized.

The ear

3. *Synopsis 5–6; Scott-Brown 1/1/11*
  a. False Both are formed in membrane. The other two
          elements of the temporal bone are the styloid process
          (derived from cartilage of the second arch) and the
          petromastoid (formed in cartilage).
  b. True The incomplete tympanic ring grows asymmetrically,
          leaving a deficiency in the external canal antero-
          inferiorly, and so infection may spread between
          parotid and meatus.
  c. False It is the thick middle layer of the petromastoid
          (enchondral layer) that may undergo defective
          ossification, particularly anterior to the oval window, a
          frequent site of otosclerotic foci.
  d. False The mastoid is flat at birth and the stylomastoid
          foramen through which the facial nerve emerges is
          very superficial, so it is at risk from injury.
  e. False It lies above, and is only 2 mm deep – hence the
          increased risk to the facial nerve and labyrinth
          during surgery.

4. *Synopsis 6–8; Scott-Brown 1/1/26*
  a. False In the diploic type the air cells are small with little
          marrow space.
  b. True However, this theory is not supported by evidence.
  c. True.
  d. True Tumarkin's theory – failure of aeration due to
          Eustachian tube blockage. Distraction theory – the
          inner and outer plates of the mastoid are separated by
          muscle pull.
  e. False 80 per cent are pneumatized; 20 per cent are diploic or
          sclerotic.

5. **Anatomy of the external ear:**
   a. The auricular skin is loosely adherent to the underlying perichondrium of yellow elastic cartilage.
   b. The external meatus has the temporomandibular joint as an anterior relation, the mastoid antrum posterosuperiorly and the middle cranial fossa superiorly.
   c. The great auricular (C1 and 2), the vagus and the trigeminal nerves supply sensation.
   d. The blood supply is from branches of the external carotid artery.
   e. The lymphatics of the lobule drain to the external jugular lymph nodes.

6. **In the adult:**
   a. The external meatus is 25 mm long, and the bony inner two-thirds is directed medially and inferiorly.
   b. The bony portion of the external meatus is lined by skin bearing ceruminous glands and hairs.
   c. The yellow elastic cartilage of the outer one-third of the meatus is deficient superiorly.
   d. Skin lining the bony meatus is closely adherent at the tympanomastoid and squamotympanic sutures.
   e. The pain of meatal furunculosis is due to a mild osteitis.

5. *Synopsis 8–9; Scott-Brown 1/1/12–14, 3/6/10–16, 3/13/2*
   a. False The skin is very closely adherent; hence the extreme pain of haematomata and the oedema of external otitis. This skin is loosely adherent in the region of the mastoid, a donor site for full thickness skin graft.
   b. True Condylar movements may be conducted to the cartilaginous meatus (Costen's syndrome).
   c. False The great auricular nerve is C2 and 3 (posterior surface pinna); the vagus (Arnold's nerve) – posterior meatus; trigeminal (V3 auriculotemporal) – anterior meatus. There is probably some supply to the concha from the facial nerve, as evidenced by the site of vesicular eruption in herpes zoster.
   d. True The auriculotemporal branch of the superficial temporal artery and the posterior auricular artery are ultimately derived from the external carotid artery.
   e. True.

6. *Synopsis 8–9, 84; Scott-Brown 1/1/12–14*
   a. True The bony meatus is also narrower than the cartilaginous portion.
   b. False Only the skin lining the cartilaginous portion of the meatus contains these structures.
   c. True The defect is between the lamina of the tragus and the crus of the helix, and is exploited in the endaural incision.
   d. True This fact, plus the thinness of the skin, makes elevation of a tympanomeatal flap difficult in these areas.
   e. False The skin is closely adherent in the cartilaginous portion (hair follicle-bearing area), leaving little room for expansion.

7. **In the middle ear cleft:**
   a. The lining is pseudo-stratified columnar ciliated epithelium anteriorly, but flat or cuboidal posteriorly.
   b. The Eustachian tube is 37 mm long, the upper two-thirds consisting of bone and the lower one-third of an incomplete ring of cartilage.
   c. Active contraction of the tensor palati results in the nasopharyngeal orifice of the Eustachian tube opening.
   d. Due to the Eustachian tube's shorter length, wider diameter and relatively more horizontal alignment in the infant, the risk of ascending infection is increased.
   e. The Eustachian tube is actively closed by the action of the palatal muscles.

8. **The anterior wall of the tympanic cavity:**
   a. This contains the notch of Rivinus.
   b. It is the site of the Glasserian fissure containing the tympanic artery and anterior ligament of the malleus.
   c. The chorda tympani, supplying light touch and proprioception to the anterior two-thirds of the tongue, leaves through the canal of Hugier.
   d. It contains the root of the processus cochleariformis, round which passes the tensor tympani muscle.
   e. It is perforated by caroticotympanic nerves and by the tympanic artery.

7. *Synopsis 10–14, 112–114; Scott-Brown 1/1/15–26, 3/3/1–3, 3/3/19, 3/10/1–2*
    a. True This difference may explain the different pathological processes seen in chronic suppurative otitis media (cuboidal region – atticoantral cholesteatoma; columnar region – tubotympanic mucosal inflammation, polyps and granulations).
    b. False The upper one-third is bone and the lower two-thirds cartilage. The cartilaginous deficiency is bridged by fibrous connective tissue.
    c. True The tensor palati takes its origin from the lateral aspect of the cartilaginous part of the Eustachian tube. The levator palati also acts to open the tube.
    d. True.
    e. False In the inactive or resting phase, the Eustachian tube is closed passively.

8. *Synopsis 10–14; Scott-Brown 1/1/15–26*
    a. False This notch is the region where the pars flaccida is attached to the squamous portion of the temporal bone superiorly (the tympanic incisura).
    b. True Also called the petrotympanic suture, the Glasserian fissure connects the middle ear and temporomandibular and parotid regions. It is a potential route for the spread of infection.
    c. False The chorda tympani does exit via the canal of Hugier, but carries only taste fibres from the anterior two-thirds of the tongue.
    d. True It is an important landmark for the first genu of the facial nerve.
    e. True The nerves are derived from the sympathetic plexus on the internal carotid artery sheath.

9. **In the middle ear cleft:**
   a. The tegmen tympani is a thin plate of petrous bone separating the cleft from the middle cranial fossa.
   b. The facial recess lies deep to the vertical portion of the facial nerve canal.
   c. The stapedius tendon is inserted into the head of the stapes.
   d. The superficial landmark of the mastoid antrum is the suprameatal triangle.
   e. The short process of the incus is attached by ligaments to the floor of the aditus.

10. **The mucosal folds, compartments and ligaments of the middle ear cleft:**
    a. These may limit infection.
    b. The pouch of Prussak lies between the neck of the malleus and pars flaccida.
    c. The posterior ligament of the incus connects the short process of the incus to the fossa incudis.
    d. The lateral ligament of the malleus is attached to the margin of the tympanic notch of Rivinus.
    e. The pouches of Von Troltsch lie between the malleolar folds and the handle of the malleus.

11. **The middle ear cleft:**
    a. The tegmen tympani and antri separate the middle ear cleft from the posterior cranial fossa.
    b. The horizontal and vertical portions of the facial nerve always traverse in bony canals.
    c. The Vth and VIth cranial nerves may be affected by spreading middle ear disease.
    d. The jugular bulb may be located in the mesotympanum.
    e. The sigmoid portion of the lateral sinus is posteromedial to the mastoid process.

9. *Synopsis 10–14; Scott-Brown 1/1/15–26*
    a. True   It is continuous with the tegmen antri.
    b. False The sinus tympani lies deep to it, and may form a site
              for hidden cholesteatoma. The facial recess lies lateral
              to the vertical facial canal, but deep to the tympanic
              annulus.
    c. False It is inserted into the neck.
    d. True   This is otherwise called MacEwen's triangle, and the
              antrum is approximately 1.5 cm deep to it in the adult.
    e. True   The short process serves as a landmark for the
              horizontal semicircular canal (which is medial to it)
              and the facial nerve (which is inferomedial).

10. *Synopsis 13; Scott-Brown 1/1/23*
    a. True.
    b. True.
    c. True.
    d. True.
    e. True   The anterior pouch is between the anterior malleolar
              fold and tympanic membrane anterior to the handle.
              The posterior pouch is between the posterior malleolar
              fold and tympanic membrane posterior to the handle.

11. *Synopsis 10–14, 117; Scott-Brown 1/1/15–20, 3/12/1–22*
    a. False They separate the cleft from the middle cranial fossa
              and, hence, the temporal lobe. Deficiency of the
              tegmen, or its erosion by cholesteatoma, may lead to
              intracranial complications of otitis media.
    b. False Bony coverings may be thin or dehiscent; thus there is
              a greater risk to the nerve during surgery and otitis
              media.
    c. True   Gradenigo's syndrome (ipsilateral facial pain, lateral
              rectus palsy and otorrhoea).
    d. True   This may occur if the tympanic cavity floor is
              dehiscent. It may be at risk during myringotomy.
    e. True   Hence the occasional spread of disease of the middle
              cleft, leading to lateral sinus thrombophlebitis and
              otitic hydrocephalus.

12. **The neurovascular supply of the middle ear cleft:**
    a. The hypotympanum is supplied by the inferior tympanic artery.
    b. The internal carotid artery supplies the anterior mesotympanum.
    c. The postauricular artery supplies the mastoid air cells.
    d. Sensation is derived from the glossopharyngeal nerve.
    e. Both the vagus and cochleovestibular nerves give a motor supply to middle ear muscles.

13. **The anatomy of the labyrinth:**
    a. The orifice of the vestibular aqueduct is located in the anterior part of the medial wall of the bony vestibule.
    b. The most superior part of the superior semicircular canal is located beneath the arcuate eminence.
    c. In the anatomical position, the plane of the lateral semicircular canals is at an angle of 30° to the horizontal, tilting down posteriorly.
    d. The osseous labyrinth contains endolymph and the membranous labyrinth perilymph.
    e. The scala media is also known as the cochlear duct.

14. **In the inner ear:**
    a. The scala tympani, containing endolymph, communicates with the subarachnoid space via the cochlear aqueduct.
    b. Cortilymph is similar to perilymph.
    c. There are three to four rows of outer hair cells, which are arranged in rows in a pattern of a 'W'.
    d. The inner hair cells are columnar in shape compared to the outer hair cells, which are bulbous.
    e. The stria vascularis is located on the outer aspect of the cochlear duct.

The ear

12. *Synopsis 14, 25; Scott-Brown 1/1/22–24, 3/13/1*
  a. True The artery is a branch of the ascending pharyngeal artery, which is the second branch of the external carotid.
  b. True The supply is via a branch called the ramus tympanici, which pierces the anterior wall.
  c. True The supply is via its stylomastoid branch.
  d. True This is via Jacobson's branch to the tympanic plexus; hence referred otalgia from lesions of the posterior one-third of the tongue.
  e. False The trigeminal nerve supplies the tensor tympani muscle, and the facial nerve (nerve to stapedius) supplies the stapedius muscle.

13. *Synopsis 15–18, 76, 132; Scott-Brown 1/1/28–44, 1/4/38, 2/21/19–20, 3/14/19, 3/21/22*
  a. False It is located in the posterior wall, and so lies on the posterior of the petrous bone. The aqueduct contains the endolymphatic duct and a small vein.
  b. True This provides an important surgical landmark in the middle fossa approach.
  c. True The patient is therefore placed supine with the head tilted 30° upwards to perform caloric tests. This position brings the lateral canals into a vertical plane, most sensitive to a thermal gradient.
  d. False The reverse is true. A perilymph leak may be produced by opening the bony labyrinth, for example at stapedectomy, or rupture of the round window membrane.
  e. False It is the portion of the membranous labyrinth containing endolymph.

14. *Synopsis 16–22, 147; Scott-Brown 1/1/28–44, 3/1/3, 3/14/25–27, 3/17/54*
  a. False It contains perilymph. The intracranial communication is correct and may be the route of pressure transmission from cranium to the inner ear, leading to round window ruptures.
  b. True It may be derived from the scala tympani via foramina in the osseous spiral lamina.
  c. True.
  d. False The reverse is true.
  e. True.

15. **In the cochlear nerve:**
    a. The type I fibres are efferent and type II afferent.
    b. The cell bodies of the afferent nerves are located in the spiral ganglion.
    c. The first synapse is at the dorsal and ventral cochlear nuclei, after which the majority of fibres ascend in the contralateral lateral lemniscus.
    d. The primary auditory centres are located in the trapezoid body.
    e. The olivocochlear fibres are type II fibres, originate from both olivary nuclei and terminate at the base of the cochlea.

16. **In the vestibular labyrinth:**
    a. The three semicircular ducts open into the utricle via six separate openings.
    b. The utriculo-endolymphatic valve consists of flaps of mucosa permitting inflow but not outflow of endolymph.
    c. The macula of the utricle lies in the horizontal plane and that of the saccule in a vertical plane.
    d. The hair cells of the utricular macula project into a membrane containing otoliths.
    e. Depolarization of a sensory cell occurs if the sensory hairs are displaced away from the kinocilium.

17. **The vestibular nerve:**
    a. Scarpa's ganglion is located in the internal auditory canal.
    b. There are anastamotic connections between the superior vestibular nerve and facial nerve.
    c. The inferior vestibular nerve supplies the posterior canal and the saccule.
    d. The vestibular nuclei send fibres to the medial longitudinal bundle (MLB), and these are responsible for reflex postural muscle tone.
    e. The blood supply is mainly from the internal auditory artery, which is derived from the posterior inferior cerebellar artery.

15. *Synopsis 18–20; Scott-Brown 1/1/39–49, 2/18/2–4*
a. False Type I fibres (23–40 000) are sparsely granulated and afferent. Type II fibres (500–600) are richly granulated, efferent, and originate in the superior olivary nucleus.
b. True.
c. True.
d. False They are located in the pons (medial geniculate body and inferior colliculus).
e. True One-fifth of the fibres are homolateral; four-fifths are contralateral. These olivocochlear fibres are probably responsible for fine tuning the cochlea, and have been implicated in the production of otoacoustic emissions and tinnitus.

16. *Synopsis 20–22; Scott-Brown 1/1/28–38, 1/4/3–11, 3/5/1–13*
a. False There are only five openings, as the posterior and superior canals have a common crus into the utricle.
b. False The valvular action is produced by the acute angle formed as the endolymphatic duct leaves the utricle.
c. True The macula is sensory epithelium, and in the semicircular canals is represented by the crista of each ampulla.
d. True The hair cells are embedded in the statoconial membrane, which contains calcite particles (statoconia).
e. False This causes hyperpolarization and a reduction in firing rate of vestibular nerve fibres.

17. *Synopsis 22, 162; Scott-Brown 1/1/41–43, 3/5/4, 3/18/10, 3/19/32*
a. True In a vestibular neurectomy the transection should be sited proximal to the ganglion, otherwise there is a risk of regeneration of nerve fibres.
b. True Connections are via the nerve of Oort.
c. True The posterior ampullary branch can be sectioned (Gacek's singular neurectomy) for treatment of the severe protracted form of benign paroxysmal positional vertigo. It is approached by drilling below the round window membrane. Alternatively, the posterior semicircular canal can be occluded.
d. False Vestibular fibres to the MLB influence the third, fourth and sixth nerve nuclei and, hence, the extrinsic ocular muscles. The vestibulospinal tract is responsible for muscle tone.
e. False The internal auditory artery is a branch of the anterior inferior cerebellar artery, but may arise directly from the basilar artery.

18. **Blood supply of the labyrinth:**
    a. The internal auditory artery divides into anterior vestibular and common cochlear branches.
    b. The cochlear artery ultimately forms the stria vascularis.
    c. The spiral modiolar artery has rich anastomoses with terminal branches of the vestibulocochlear artery.
    d. The vestibulocochlear artery is a branch of the common cochlear artery.
    e. The labyrinthine artery is the principal arterial supply of the inner ear.

19. **Anatomy of the internal auditory canal:**
    a. The fundus, at the lateral end, is a vertical plate of thin solid bone.
    b. The transverse crest separates the inferior vestibular nerve from the cochlear nerve.
    c. 'Bill's' bar, or the vertical crest, was named after King William IV of England.
    d. The vertical crest divides the upper compartment into an anterior portion for the facial nerve and a posterior portion for the superior vestibular nerve.
    e. The foramen singulare in the lower compartment transmits the nerve from the posterior semicircular canal.

18. *Synopsis 23, 162; Scott-Brown 1/1/43–44, 3/5/16, 3/10/10, 3/17/12–17*
    a. True The internal auditory artery is usually derived from the anterior inferior cerebellar artery, but may arise directly from the basilar artery.
    b. True The stria vascularis is probably the site of both formation and absorption of endolymph and hence the source of electrical potentials in the inner ear.
    c. False The spiral modiolar artery is an end artery, and obstruction to its blood flow is a potential cause of sudden sensorineural deafness.
    d. True.
    e. True This is also called the internal auditory artery.

19. *Synopsis 23–24; Scott-Brown 1/1/27, 3/18/10, 3/21/22–28*
    a. False The plate contains numerous perforations that transmit the fibres of the vestibulocochlear and facial nerves.
    b. False It divides the internal auditory canal into a small upper compartment (facial and superior vestibular nerves) and a larger lower compartment (cochlear and inferior vestibular nerves).
    c. False It is named after William House, of the House Ear Institute, Los Angeles.
    d. True.
    e. True This nerve is occasionally sectioned in persistent severe cases of benign paroxysmal positional vertigo (singular neurectomy).

20. **Sensory nerve supply of the ear:**
    a. The lesser occipital nerve (C1) supplies the upper medial surface of the pinna.
    b. The 'Alderman's nerve' may be stimulated by instilling spirit or instruments into the external meatus.
    c. The glossopharyngeal nerve supplies sensory fibres to the middle ear cleft.
    d. The mandibular nerve supplies sensation to the lateral surface of the pinna and the anterior halves of the external meatus and tympanic membrane.
    e. The VIIth cranial nerve gives a sensory supply to the ear.

21. **The following lesions may cause referred otalgia:**
    a. Fibrositis of the upper portion of the sternomastoid muscle via the fibres of C2 and C3.
    b. A high septal deviation causing pressure on the middle turbinate.
    c. Parotid and submandibular calculi.
    d. Acute sphenoidal and maxillary sinusitis.
    e. An elongated styloid process.

20. *Synopsis 25; Scott-Brown 1/1/13,17, 3/1/1, 3/13/1, 5/20/17, 6/33/5–7*
  a. False The area supplied is correct, but the lesser occipital is derived from C2. C1 has no sensory fibres. Referred otalgia via this nerve may occur in pathologies of the cervical vertebrae.
  b. True This is also called Arnold's nerve (auricular branch of the vagus). Instrumentation occasionally causes coughing paroxysms. The nerve supplies the posterior half of the external meatus and tympanic membrane. Instillation of spirit is said to enhance the appetite by reflex vagal stimulation, and was carried out by aldermen to increase their capacity for banqueting.
  c. True This is via the tympanic plexus derived from the tympanic branch of the glossopharyngeal nerve. It is the site of tympanic neurectomy for gustatory sweating occurring after parotid surgery.
  d. True Supply is via its auriculotemporal branch. It is hence a cause of referred otalgia produced by petrous apex pathology (acoustic nerve tumours, primary cholesteatoma etc.), which irritates the trigeminal nerve.
  e. True This is based on the earache and conchal lesions produced by herpes zoster oticus (Ramsay Hunt syndrome).

21. *Synopsis 25–26; Scott-Brown 3/1/1, 3/13/1–8*
  a. True.
  b. True Transmission is via the trigeminal nerve. This pathology may also give rise to facial pain.
  c. True Transmission is via the trigeminal nerve.
  d. True Transmission is via the trigeminal nerve.
  e. True This stretches the glossopharyngeal nerve as it routes round the process, and causes stabbing pain in the side of the oropharynx and ear during mastication. The styloid process can usually be palpated in the tonsillar fossa, and is readily visualized on plain X-rays.

22. **The following neoplasms may present with otalgia:**
    a. Nasopharyngeal carcinoma.
    b. Tonsillar carcinoma.
    c. Oesophageal carcinoma.
    d. Oropharyngeal carcinoma.
    e. Chemodectoma of the larynx.

23. **Clinical examination of the ear:**
    a. The normal tympanic membrane is blue in colour.
    b. Mobility of the eardrum can be assessed with Siegle's speculum.
    c. The pars flaccida is also known clinically as the 'attic'.
    d. Pneumatic otoscopy is helpful in differentiating a perforation from a retraction pocket.
    e. Examination of the nasopharyngeal end of the Eustachian tube should be routine in the presence of an effusion.

22. *Synopsis 24–26; Scott-Brown 3/1/1, 3/13/1–8, 5/11/8, 5/13/12, 5/14/8*
- a. True Otalgia is caused by ulceration and invasion of the mandibular division of the trigeminal as it emerges through the foramen ovale.
- b. True There may be referred otalgia via the glossopharyngeal nerve.
- c. True This is rare. Otalgia occurs via the vagus nerve, particularly if the lesion has involved the recurrent laryngeal nerve coursing in the tracheo-oesophageal groove. Pharyngeal neoplasia causes referred otalgia early in its evolution.
- d. True This is via the glossopharyngeal and vagus nerves.
- e. True This is an unusual tumour, and causes severe local pain and referred otalgia.

23. *Synopsis 26–28; Scott-Brown 3/1/5–9*
- a. False It is normally light grey, but is commonly blue in cases of glue ear, haemotympanum, high jugular bulb and cholesterol granuloma.
- b. True It may also be assessed using a pneumatic attachment to an electric auriscope. The Valsalva and Toynbee manoeuvres are also useful tests of mobility and Eustachian tube function.
- c. True Although 'attic' is the most frequently used term for this region, it is strictly that part of the middle ear cleft above the pars flaccida. Epitympanum and attic are synonyms.
- d. True The drum will not move very much with pressure changes if there is a perforation. The retraction pocket may evert when a negative pressure is applied to the meatus.
- e. True It can be viewed with a mirror, flexible fibreoptic nasolaryngoscope or rigid nasal endoscope.

24. Imaging of the temporal bone:
    a. Plain X-ray films of the mastoids are the most useful investigation in suspected chronic suppurative otitis media (CSOM).
    b. High-resolution CT scanning in the axial plane allows accurate differential characterization of soft tissue abnormalities.
    c. Digital subtraction angiography (DSA) is more hazardous than direct puncture arteriography.
    d. Magnetic resonance imaging is the most useful investigation in suspected acoustic neuroma.
    e. Computerized tomography in the coronal plane can display the descending facial nerve canal well, but results in unacceptably high radiation exposure levels to the eye.

25. The following procedures are usually performed via a permeatal incision:
    a. Exploration of the vertical portion of the facial nerve.
    b. Membranous labyrinthectomy for Ménière's disease.
    c. Tympanic neurectomy.
    d. Cochlear implantation.
    e. Fenestration of the lateral semicircular canal.

24. *Synopsis 28–31; Scott-Brown 3/2/1–38*

  a. False   CSOM is a clinical diagnosis made on the basis of
                history and examination, preferably under the
                operating microscope. In cases where imaging is
                deemed necessary, plain X-rays have been almost
                entirely superseded by sectional imaging techniques.
  b. False   Although CT is excellent at showing intracranial
                complications and bony anatomy, soft tissue
                differentiation remains poor.
  c. False   DSA is safer, and provides information almost as
                detailed as traditional arteriography. MR angiography
                is also rapidly advancing.
  d. True   This can demonstrate very tiny lesions accurately.
  e. False   The descending facial nerve canal can be demonstrated
                well, and orbital radiation exposure is less from
                coronal than from axial cuts.

25. *Synopsis 32, 35; Scott-Brown 3/19/36, 3/24/27–28, 3/25/10*

  a. False   Only the horizontal portion of the facial nerve is seen
                in this approach. A postauricular or endaural approach
                will allow exposure of the vertical portion.
  b. True   This is carried out by turning the stapes with its
                footplate laterally, hooking out the saccule and
                instilling a vestibulotoxic agent to destroy any
                remaining neuroepithelium.
  c. True   This may be carried out in severe cases of gustatory
                sweating after parotid surgery (Frey's syndrome) that
                do not resolve spontaneously. It has been advocated for
                reduction of drooling in cerebral palsy. As with other
                forms of autonomic surgery, the results are reasonably
                good initially but rarely last longer than 2 years.
  d. False   An extended postauricular incision, entering the
                middle ear via a posterior tympanotomy is the usual
                approach.
  e. False   This has become an obsolete operation for otosclerosis
                since the introduction of stapedectomy. It was usually
                carried out via Lempert's endaural approach.

26. **In temporal bone surgery:**
    a. The suprameatal triangle is the surface landmark of the mastoid antrum.
    b. The endaural incision divides tragal cartilage at the incisura terminalis.
    c. All postaural incisions should be placed about 1 cm behind the postauricular sulcus and extend inferiorly to the tip of the mastoid process.
    d. Trautmann's triangle is part of the bony plate of the posterior cranial fossa.
    e. The bone over an infant's antrum is microscopically cribriform.

27. **Principles of temporal bone surgery:**
    a. The radical mastoidectomy involves complete removal of the ossicles and tympanic membrane and lowering of the posterior canal wall.
    b. In an attico-antrostomy, the only ossicle removed is the incus.
    c. In combined approach tympanoplasty (canal wall up mastoidectomy), access to the mesotympanum is obtained via anterior tympanotomy and directly via the external meatus.
    d. The solid angle is formed by bone in the angle between the three semicircular canals.
    e. In a Schwartze cortical mastoidectomy, the posterior canal wall is lowered.

28. **Course of the facial nerve through the temporal bone:**
    a. The narrowest part of the fallopian canal is at the entrance from the internal auditory meatus.
    b. The nerve normally lies deep to the short process of the incus.
    c. At the second genu, the nerve normally lies deep to the pyramidal process.
    d. The anterior end of the digastric ridge is a useful landmark for the stylomastoid foramen.
    e. The processus cochleariformis is a landmark for the geniculate ganglion, which lies superior to it.

26. *Synopsis 32–38; Scott-Brown 3/9/9, 3/10/6*
  a. True   In an adult the mastoid antrum is located 1.5 cm deep to the landmark, which is also called MacEwen's triangle.
  b. False No cartilage is divided, hence there is a reduced risk of perichondritis.
  c. False In infants and young children the inferior extension should not extend below the level of the external auditory meatus, in order to avoid damage to the superficially placed facial nerve. The mastoid process does not appear until the second year of life.
  d. True   It is bounded posteriorly by the sigmoid sinus, anteriorly by the bony labyrinth (posterior semicircular canal) and superiorly by the superior petrosal sinus.
  e. True   Therefore, an acute otitis media is actually a subperiosteal infection.

27. *Synopsis 33–38; Scott-Brown 3/9/9, 3/10/6, 3/11/2, 6/8/16–21*
  a. False The stapes footplate, with or without the superstructure, is preserved.
  b. False Both the incus and malleus head are removed.
  c. False Access is obtained via posterior tympanotomy, in the angle between the corda tympani and the descending facial nerve canal.
  d. True   It is medial to the mastoid antrum.
  e. False Wide exenteration of all mastoid air cells is performed, but the canal wall is left intact.

28. *Synopsis 36–38; Scott-Brown 3/24/6–28*
  a. True   The nerve diameter averages 0.68 mm; this is a 'bottleneck', and the commonest site for compression in inflammatory conditions.
  b. True   This provides an important landmark in temporal bone surgery.
  c. False The nerve is superficial (lateral) and posterior to the pyramid, which houses the stapedius muscle. The branch to stapedius arises on the deep surface of the facial nerve.
  d. True.
  e. True   This provides another important landmark in temporal bone surgery.

29. **Physical properties of sound:**
    a. Frequency is subjectively perceived as pitch.
    b. A hearing loss of 60 dB means that sounds have to be one million times more intense than the normal threshold to be heard.
    c. The reference intensity pressure in audiometry is 0.024 dyne/cm^2 at 100 Hz.
    d. Overtones are multiples of the fundamental note.
    e. Free field measurements of sound intensity are usually calibrated in the physical dB-SPL scale, which is not directly comparable with pure tone audiometers calibrated in the biological dB-HL scale.

30. **Sound transmission in the middle ear:**
    a. The intact tympanic membrane protects the round window and directs sound energy to the ossicular chain and oval window.
    b. The ossicular leverage action ratio of the malleus and incus is about 1.3:1.
    c. The mode of vibration of the stapes changes with high sound intensities.
    d. The physiological ratio of tympanic membrane to oval window surface area is about 21:1.
    e. The transformer ratio of the ossicular chain plus the tympanic membrane is about 18:1.

31. **Pathological states causing conductive deafness:**
    a. Increased stiffness caused by adhesions and tympanosclerosis have a greater effect on low frequencies.
    b. The presence of fluid in the middle ear affects mainly the high frequencies.
    c. Ossicular chain discontinuity with an intact tympanic membrane results in reduced middle ear compliance.
    d. Posterior perforations cause a greater hearing loss than similar-sized anterior perforations.
    e. Tympanosclerosis increases the middle ear compliance.

29. *Synopsis 39–40; Scott-Brown 1/2/1–6, 1/3/11, 3/1/15*
  a. True.
  b. True Subjective loudness has a logarithmic relationship to physical sound intensity.
  c. False It is 0.00024 dyne/cm^2 at 1000 Hz.
  d. True They are subjectively perceived as quality or timbre. The fundamental note is the frequency of the lowest note.
  c. True The equivalent dB-HL is up to 11 dB less than the dB-SPL, depending on the frequency tested.

30. *Synopsis 41–45; Scott-Brown 1/2/6–14*
  a. True Sound energy is preferentially transmitted to the oval window. The eardrum acts as a baffle, preventing sound reaching the round window.
  b. True The axis of rotation is a line joining the anterior process of the malleus and short process of the incus.
  c. True With low intensity sounds, the axis is near the posterior margin of the footplate. At high intensity, the axis runs longitudinally through the footplate. The latter affords greater protection of the delicate inner ear structures.
  d. False The anatomical ratio is 21:1, but the tympanic membrane is fixed at its periphery so only two-thirds is available for physiological vibration. Therefore, the physiological ratio is about 14:1.
  e. True This allows some degree of impedance matching between the external air and inner ear fluids.

31. *Synopsis 42–44; Scott-Brown 1/2/12–13*
  a. True Changes in stiffness mainly affect the lower frequencies.
  b. False The low frequencies are mainly affected, due to increased stiffness (reduced compliance).
  c. False The compliance is increased.
  d. True This is because the round window is exposed, reducing the differential sound pressure between oval and round windows.
  e. False It reduces compliance by increasing the stiffness of the vibrating parts.

32. **Abnormalities of middle ear function:**
    a.   Loss of the transformer mechanism alone produces a hearing loss of about 50 dB.
    b.   A round window baffle effect in modified radical mastoidectomy may allow a hearing threshold within 25 dB of normal.
    c.   A columellar effect is produced by conservation of only the ossicular chain lever ratio of the transformer mechanism.
    d.   No sound is perceived by air conduction if there is total loss of the middle ear mechanism.
    e.   A blast injury may increase middle ear compliance.

33. **Middle ear muscles:**
    a.   Reflex contraction of the stapedius to sound stimulus is ipsilateral.
    b.   Contractions may be audible.
    c.   The tensor tympani pulls the tympanic membrane medially and stiffens the ossicular chain.
    d.   Contraction attenuates the middle and high frequencies.
    e.   Contraction allows protection against acoustic trauma due to explosions.

34. **Hearing by bone conduction:**
    a.   Bone conduction is the normal physiological route for hearing one's own voice.
    b.   Tonndorf's experiments implied there may be a physiological 'third window' in the cochlea, via the cochlear aqueduct and blood vessels.
    c.   This is used as a measure of cochlear function.
    d.   Movement of the cochlear fluids because of differential distortion of the large scala vestibuli compared to the small scala tympani is known as the distortional vibration factor.
    e.   Shunting of pressure changes via a normal oval window, compared with enhancement by a stiff ossicular chain, may explain lateralization of the Weber test to the ear with the conductive hearing loss.

32. *Synopsis 42–44; Scott-Brown 1/2/12*
  a. False   The loss is only 25–30 dB (round window protection is maintained).
  b. True   Although the transformer mechanism is lost, the preferential sound conduction to the oval windows is maintained. Hence there is only a 25 dB loss instead of the expected 40–60 dB loss.
  c. False   The ossicular chain lever ratio is lost, and the area ratio of the drumhead and oval window preserved.
  d. False   The basilar membrane moves due to yielding of the inner ear contents.
  e. True   This may occur if ossicular disconnection has occurred.

33. *Synopsis 13,44; Scott-Brown 1/1/21, 1/2/11–12*
  a. False   The reflex is consensual.
  b. True   This is particularly true of the tensor tympani, giving a rare cause of tinnitus.
  c. True.
  d. False   It attenuates the more damaging low frequencies, allowing preferential transmission of the middle and high frequencies.
  e. False   The latency of the muscle reflexes means that they cannot contract in time to protect against high intensity noise of sudden onset.

34. *Synopsis 44; Scott-Brown 1/2/13–14*
  a. True   Effective stimuli include the subject's own voice, ambient sound pressures and direct contact with a vibrating object (as in tuning fork tests).
  b. True   In experiments using cats, some bone conduction occurred despite sealing both round and oval windows with cement. This response was reduced by sealing the cochlear aqueduct.
  c. True   Tuning fork tests and bone conduction audiometry may be used.
  d. True.
  e. True.

35. **Cochlear physiology:**
    a. The perilymph and cerebrospinal fluid are connected by the vestibular aqueduct.
    b. The scala media has a resting electrical potential of +80 mV with reference to the scala tympani.
    c. Short travelling waves in the basilar membrane are produced by low-pitched sound stimuli.
    d. The cochlear microphonic potential is generated by the outer hair cells.
    e. A summating potential (SP) is predominantly produced by outer hair cell activity.

36. **Transduction of sound signals into electrical activity in the auditory nerve:**
    a. Movement of the basilar membrane relative to the tectorial membrane stretches transduction links between the tips of hair cell stereocilia and opens ion channels in the hair cell membrane.
    b. The outer hair cells improve frequency selectivity by a mechanical amplifying effect on basilar membrane displacement.
    c. Each inner hair cell has terminals from about 20 afferent cochlear nerve fibres.
    d. The release of neurotransmitters from the base of the inner hair cells results in action potentials in the afferent auditory nerve fibres.
    e. The highly specific tuning curves of cochlear nerve fibres depend on mechanical amplification of basilar membrane displacement by normally functioning outer hair cells.

37. **Localization of sound stimulus:**
    a. Interaural phase differences are important for low frequencies.
    b. Complex sounds and transients are detected by differences in their times of arrival at the ears.
    c. The head produces a shadow effect on sound.
    d. Monaural hearing is more efficient than binaural hearing.
    e. Interaural intensity differences are important for frequencies above 1500 Hz.

35. *Synopsis 46–49; Scott-Brown 1/1/31, 1/2/14–31*
   a. False They are connected by the cochlear aqueduct.
            Perilymph is probably a blood filtrate, and has a
            different composition to CSF.
   b. True.
   c. False The short wave has its maximum displacement
            near the basal turn of the cochlea, and is produced
            by high frequencies. Low frequencies produce a
            long travelling wave, with maximal displacement
            nearer the apex.
   d. True It is absent if the hair cells are damaged, for example
            by aminoglycosides such as streptomycin.
   e. False The SP is produced by inner hair cell activity in
            response to high frequency sound stimuli.

36. *Synopsis 48–50; Scott-Brown 1/2/17–31*
   a. True The links are arranged radially across the cochlear
            duct, making them most sensitive to the movement.
   b. True The amplifying effect is up to 40 dB at each
            specific frequency.
   c. True.
   d. True.
   e. True.

37. *Synopsis 50; Scott-Brown 1/2/15–16*
   a. True They are important below 1500 Hz.
   b. True.
   c. True This is particularly so with high frequencies, and thus
            produces interaural intensity differences.
   d. False.
   e. True.

38. **Testing the hearing:**
    a. The 1024 Hz tuning fork is best for general use.
    b. Masking the good ear in severe unilateral sensorineural deafness is essential.
    c. The Weber test always lateralizes to the better ear in sensorineural deafness.
    d. The Stenger test is a test to detect a feigned unilateral hearing loss, where two tones of different frequencies but the same intensity are presented to each ear simultaneously.
    e. In normal ears, the Rinne test is usually neutral.

39. **In non-organic hearing loss:**
    a. Electrocochleography (ECochG) is essential to detect any thresholds.
    b. The stapedial reflex is seldom of value.
    c. Serial audiograms are usually inconsistent.
    d. The Chimani-Moos test is a modification of the Weber test.
    e. The Stenger test can be performed either with two tuning forks or an audiometer.

38. *Synopsis 51–52; Scott-Brown 2/5/1–6, 3/1/8–11*
   a. False   The 512 Hz tuning fork is most useful. Below 256 Hz
         the vibrations are felt rather than heard; above
         1024 Hz they fade too rapidly.
   b. True   If it is not masked, a false negative Rinne may be
         elicited; hence the use of a Barany box. Masking is
         essential during audiometric threshold assessment.
   c. False   This may not occur in long-standing sensorineural
         deafness.
   d. False   The tones are of same frequency but different
         intensity, the alleged deaf ear being presented with a
         louder sound than the good ear. A patient with a true
         unilateral hearing loss will still hear the quieter sound
         in the opposite ear, whereas the malingerer will deny
         hearing any sound at all.
   e. False   In normal ears it is positive, AC better than BC.

39. *Synopsis 51–62; Scott-Brown 2/4/7, 2/5/5–6, 2/12/14–15,*
   2/12/21–24, 3/1/11, 3/1/24–26
   a. False   Thresholds can be estimated without any electrical
         tests. The non-invasive brainstem-evoked response
         (BSER) and the cortical electrical response
         audiometry (CERA) are more widely used than
         ECochG.
   b. False   This is a useful objective test, provided it is used in
         conjunction with other audiological investigations.
   c. True   A shadow audiogram of an unmasked 'good' ear is also
         rarely produced. In a genuine case, the shadow
         audiogram would be expected with stimuli in excess of
         50 dB applied to the deaf ear.
   d. True   The malingerer hears the tuning fork in the good ear,
         and may say that nothing is heard when the same ear is
         occluded.
   e. True   The principle is that two tones of equal frequency
         cannot both be heard if one is louder than the other.

40. Audiological investigations:
  a. Masking for air conduction is necessary if the hearing loss of the test ear exceeds 50 dB.
  b. A retrocochlear deafness gives a speech discrimination far better than expected from pure tone thresholds.
  c. In Bekesy audiometry, a sweep of frequencies is presented automatically by the machine, the subject is asked to control the intensity (keeping the sound at a just audible level), and the result is plotted automatically.
  d. Recruitment is an abnormally increased subjective sensation of loudness for a given increase in intensity, is characteristic of cochlear pathology, and can be tested for by the Fowler alternate binaural loudness balance test.
  e. Masking is essential for bone conduction thresholds because the interaural attenuation for bone-conducted sound is less than 5 dB.

41. Impedance audiometry (tympanometry):
  a. The standard tympanometer probe produces a tone of 220 Hz at 85 dB-SPL, and a pressure range of approximately –200 to +200 dPa.
  b. The peak of the tympanometry curve corresponds to the point at which the tympanic membrane is most freely mobile, and is a good estimate of middle ear pressure.
  c. A flat tympanogram (Jerger type B) means glue ear.
  d. The ipsilateral acoustic reflex depends on the functional integrity of the facial nerve branch to stapedius, and on normal mobility of the middle ear structures.
  e. An impedance value of over 2 ml on a tympanogram may indicate the presence of a perforation of the tympanic membrane with a blocked Eustachian tube.

40. *Synopsis 51–62; Scott-Brown 2/4/7, 2/12/14–15, 2/12/21–27, 3/1/11–26*
  a. True At this level, sounds may be conducted to the non-test ear by skull vibrations. Masking is necessary in all bone conduction measurements, and consists of narrow-band filtered white noise centred on the test frequency.
  b. False Classically the speech discrimination score is very poor. Cochlear deafness produces the 'rollover' effect, where the speech score deteriorates with increasing intensity levels.
  c. True This method is most commonly used in occupational health screening programmes.
  d. True Until recently, formal tests for recruitment were an important part of diagnostic audiology, in the attempt to select patients for invasive examinations such as air meatography for exclusion of acoustic neuroma. Development and wide availability of MRI scanning have reduced its diagnostic importance, but consideration of recruitment remains critical in the design and fitting of hearing aids.
  e. True.

41. *Synopsis 57–60; Scott-Brown 2/12/12–17, 3/1/20–23*
  a. True.
  b. True.
  c. False A flat tympanogram does occur in glue ear, but could also mean that the probe opening was blocked due to wax or faulty technique.
  d. True This explains its diagnostic value in assessing the level of a facial nerve lesion.
  e. True The same measurement may be obtained with a patent grommet, but only if the Eustachian tube is blocked. This figure is the compliance value of the whole middle ear cleft.

42. **Electric response audiometry:**
    a. Enhancement of the summating potential on electrocochleography is characteristic of Ménière's disease.
    b. Interaural latency difference of the fifth wave of greater than 0.4 ms on brain stem electrical response occurs in most cases of acoustic neuroma.
    c. The postauricular myogenic responses give a very accurate measure of hearing thresholds in young children.
    d. Electrocochleography can produce responses to stimuli of 250 Hz or less.
    e. General anaesthesia affects the responses obtained during brainstem electrical stimulation.

42. *Synopsis 60–62; Scott-Brown 2/12/21–27, 2/17/10–12, 3/1/24–26, 3/19/22*

   a. True The SP may be larger than the action potential, and the cochlear microphonic may also be abnormal.

   b. True This test was, until recently, used as part of a screening battery to select patients with unilateral sensorineural hearing loss for further radiological investigation. The widespread availability and high diagnostic sensitivity and specificity of MRI, and the realization that cases will be missed on screening protocols, now means that most patients will be sent direct for a scan on clinical suspicion alone.

   c. False A positive response merely indicates the integrity of the neural pathway.

   d. False Stimuli below 1000 Hz produce poor responses and are unreliable.

   e. False Responses are not affected by sedatives or general anaesthesia; hence its value in measuring thresholds in young or uncooperative patients or cases of suspected non-organic hearing loss.

43. Children's hearing tests and otoacoustic emissions:
   a. Distraction tests can be performed on infants below 6 months of age.
   b. Evoked otoacoustic emissions (OAE) testing is a quick, non-invasive, objective test to determine hearing thresholds accurately, and is suitable for newborn infants.
   c. Reliable pure tone audiometry (PTA) can usually be performed on subjects with a mental age of 4 years.
   d. Otoacoustic emissions show a delayed latency with increasing degrees of sensorineural hearing loss until they disappear altogether at around 85 dB-HL.
   e. Blinking, frowning and stilling are responses to sound of a normal 3-month-old child.

43. *Synopsis 62–66; Scott-Brown 3/1/26, 6/5/1–14, 6/6/1–16*
  a. False Distraction tests are useful from 6–24 months.
The stimuli employed are a high frequency rattle
(8000 Hz), a low hum (500 Hz) and a whispered 'S'
(2000–4000 Hz). An electronic device producing
warble tones is also an effective stimulus. The test
requires two people: a tester, and a 'distracter' who
engages the child's attention. Head turning occurs
toward the sound stimulus, which is presented, out of
sight of the child, at known intensities. A reasonably
accurate audiogram can be constructed in most cases.
  b. False Although OAE testing is quick, non-invasive, objective
and can be used on newborns, it does not accurately
determine thresholds. It is used as a screening test. The
presence of normal emissions means that the hearing is
likely to be normal (better than 20 dB-HL), but a failed
test may be due to anything from a very minor middle
ear problem to profound sensorineural hearing loss. The
test has a high sensitivity, but a rather poor specificity.
  c. True The mental rather than the chronological age is
important. At a mental age of 4 years, children should
be able to give reliable responses to PTA.
  d. False Otoacoustic emissions are not recordable if the hearing
loss is any greater than 20–25 dB. The latency of
auditory brainstem responses (BSERs) does increase
as the stimulus intensity is reduced.
  e. True.

44. Hearing aids:
 a. Amplification of sound by electronic hearing aids primarily improves speech discrimination in the presence of background noise.
 b. A low frequency cut may be very useful in severe high frequency losses.
 c. Vented earmoulds are useful for 'ski slope' type audiograms.
 d. Peak clipping in sensorineural hearing loss with a reduced dynamic range may lead to distortion.
 e. In standard NHS hearing aids, the switch marked 'T' is for use in the presence of an inductive loop system.

45. Vestibular labyrinthine physiology:
 a. The utricular macula responds to angular acceleration.
 b. The discharge rate of vestibular nerve fibres is zero when the subject is lying still with the head and eyes central.
 c. Ampullofugal displacement of the cupula of the superior semicircular cord increases vestibular nerve activity.
 d. The saccular maculae lie in a horizontal plane.
 e. Steady rotation is detected by the semicircular canals, even with the eyes closed.

44. *Synopsis 66–72; Scott-Brown 2/13/22–24, 2/14/1–24, 6/10/6–9*
  a. False Speech discrimination in noise is a complex function depending on intact cochlear hair cells. Simple amplification does little to address this problem, and can sometimes make it worse.
  b. True This is especially so where the low frequency energy causes loudness discomfort (recruitment). This is seen particularly in presbyacusis.
  c. True This earmould construction allows emphasis of high frequency sounds, and may give relief to the 'blocked up' feeling of a closed mould. Acoustic feedback is a problem with vented moulds.
  d. True Automatic gain control (AGC) may prevent loudness discomfort levels being reached, but there is a delay in onset of about 50 ms. However, distortion is less of a problem with AGC.
  e. True Loop systems are frequently installed in educational establishments, theatres and television sets.

45. *Synopsis 16–23, 73–75; Scott-Brown 1/1/34–42, 1/4/1–51, 1/7/25–26, 2/19/1–9*
  a. False The utricular macula lies in the horizontal plane, and therefore responds to tilt and linear acceleration.
  b. False There is steady activity, equal on both sides.
  c. True This occurs if there is ampullopetal displacement in the lateral semicircular canal.
  d. False They lie in a vertical plane, and may be concerned with the detection of low frequency vibration.
  e. False Only rotational acceleration or deceleration are detected. Constant rotational rates do not stimulate the semicircular canals.

46. **Vestibular function tests:**
    a. In the Hallpike bithermal caloric test, the ears are irrigated for 40 s with water 5°C above and below the normal body temperature.
    b. Rotation to the left indicates a labyrinthine disorder on the ipsilateral side during Unterberger's test.
    c. Computerized dynamic posturography provides an objective measurement of balance performance, and can be used to quantify improvement following surgery or vestibular rehabilitation exercises.
    d. Rotational chair testing allows the function of the right and left vestibular labyrinths to be tested separately.
    e. Electronystagmography (ENG) is more sensitive than clinical observation in the detection of rotatory nystagmus.

47. **Caloric tests:**
    a. The fixation index compares the duration of nystagmus with and without optic fixation.
    b. Bilaterally decreased responses reliably indicate peripheral labyrinthine pathology.
    c. Enhanced responses may be seen in cerebellar lesions.
    d. Frenzel's glasses abolish optic fixation.
    e. Air calorics have the advantage of being usable in the presence of a perforation of the tympanic membrane.

48. **Electronystagmography:**
    a. This measures changes in the corneovestibular electrical potentials.
    b. It may show multiple square waves in cerebellar disorders.
    c. In a normal subject, it shows smooth sinusoidal waves on pendulum eye tracking.
    d. This is unable to give a measure of the amplitude of nystagmus.
    e. It can only record nystagmus that is visible to the naked eye.

46. *Synopsis 75–80; Scott-Brown 2/21/1–35, 3/1/11–15, 3/18/5*
   a. False The irrigation time is correct, but the water temperature is 7°C above and below the normal body temperature (i.e. 44°C and 30°C).
   b. True.
   c. True The test battery involves closing the eyes to abolish visual input, and standing on a moving platform or a foam pad in order to reduce proprioceptive input.
   d. False Unless the patient's head is dehiscent in the sagittal plane, both will be rotated!
   e. False ENG is good at providing an objective record of horizontal nystagmus, but is less sensitive than clinical observation. Rotatory nystagmus may not be detected at all, because there is little or no variation in the corneo-retinal potential relative to electrode placement.

47. *Synopsis 76–78; Scott-Brown 2/21/20, 3/1/11–12, 3/18/5*
   a. True.
   b. False Decreased or absent responses may be due to habituation, e.g. in ballet dancers and acrobats.
   c. True Responses may be enhanced both in amplitude and/or in duration, usually with an ipsilateral directional preponderance.
   d. False They only reduce fixation. For complete abolition, either use Frenzel's glasses with an infrared viewer or ENG darkness for complete abolition.
   e. True They are useful in determining whether there is any vestibular function in a mastoid cavity.

48. *Synopsis 80; Scott-Brown 2/19/6, 2/21/14 18, 3/1/12*
   a. False It detects changes in the corneo-retinal potential relative to the electrode placement.
   b. True It may also reveal ocular dysmetria. On command for lateral gaze, the eyes overshoot the target.
   c. True Ataxic eye tracking movements are highly suggestive of brainstem lesions.
   d. False The ENG tracing should be calibrated before any test. It reveals both duration and amplitude of eye movements.
   e. False The advantage of ENG is that it may reveal visually undetectable nystagmus, including nystagmus that occurs on eye closure.

49. Congenital abnormalities of the external ear:
  a. Abnormalities are due to a developmental failure of the first and second elements of the branchial system.
  b. Abnormalities include collaural fistulae, which may be closely related to the glossopharyngeal nerve.
  c. 'Bat ears' (protruding ears) are associated with under-development or absence of the antihelical fold.
  d. Major deformities of the pinna are best treated with multiple-staged plastic surgical reconstruction operations.
  e. Meatal atresia is rarely associated with middle ear malformations.

50. Haematoma auris:
  a. This has vegetable connotations.
  b. It is due to extravasation of blood in the subcutaneous tissue plane.
  c. Treatment is initially by aspiration with a wide-bore needle.
  d. It should be treated by warming the pinna.
  e. It can cause loss of cartilage support of the auricle.

51. Otitis externa:
  a. Furunculosis may be misdiagnosed as acute mastoiditis.
  b. Failure to resolve can be due to employing an inappropriate topical antibiotic preparation without aural toilet.
  c. The mainstay of treating an acute infection is meatal toilet.
  d. The conidiophores of an *Aspergillus niger* fungal infection are easily identified on otoscopy.
  e. When caused by dandruff, selenium sulphide-based shampoos are beneficial.

49. *Synopsis 81–82; Scott-Brown 3/6/8–10, 3/8/1–10, 6/9/1–12*
  a. True.
  b. False They are related to the facial nerve. Congenital aural
          fistulae are lined with squamous epithelium, usually
          opening near the ascending crus of the helix.
  c. True.
  d. False These deformities are best treated by the Branemark
          titanium fixture and provision of a prosthesis.
  e. False The first arch contributes to the malleus and incus, and
          the second arch to the stapes; hence middle ear
          anomalies are quite common.

50. *Synopsis 82; Scott-Brown 3/6/4–5*
  a. True Failure to treat the blood clot results in fibrosis, with a
          deformity called a 'cauliflower ear'. It is a hazard of
          dedicated rugby forwards.
  b. False The haemorrhage is between cartilage and perichondrium.
  c. True However, this is only if the haematoma is of recent onset.
          Otherwise, a formal helical incision and suction is required.
  d. False This treatment is for frostbite of the auricle in its early
          stages, and before gangrene has supervened.
  e. True This is due to devitalization of the cartilage, or if a
          perichondritis supervenes as a result of surgical
          intervention or the haematoma becoming infected.

51. *Synopsis 83–93; Scott-Brown 3/6/6, 3/6/13–17*
  a. True This is particularly so because the former may produce
          marked meatal swelling and postauricular oedema and
          tenderness. Furunculosis may be distinguished by pain
          elicited on tragal pressure, enlargement of lymph nodes,
          postauricular tenderness (rather than over MacEwan's
          triangle) and clear mastoid air cells on X-ray.
  b. True It can also be due to underlying chronic suppurative
          otitis media, fungal superinfection, or sensitivity to the
          antibiotic preparation.
  c. True It is particularly important to remove debris in the
          anterior meatal recess.
  d. True They may be seen as black specks. After meatal toilet,
          1% clotrimazole or amphotericin cream can be applied.
  e. True In this case, the external meatus is involved in what is
          essentially a scalp condition (seborrhoeic otitis externa).

52. **Malignant otitis externa:**
    a. There is a spreading osteomyelitis of the temporal bone caused by *Haemophilus influenzae*.
    b. The parotid gland is involved by direct extension of disease.
    c. A purulent discharge coming through a tympanic perforation is commonly seen.
    d. A urinalysis is indicated.
    e. A Gradenigo syndrome may result.

53. **Viral infections of the external ear:**
    a. This may be associated with cranial nerve palsies and encephalitis.
    b. Otitis externa haemorrhagica may be associated with influenzal epidemics.
    c. Otalgia and oropharyngeal discomfort may precede the rash in herpes zoster.
    d. Aciclovir eradicates herpes infections.
    e. Bullous myringitis is characterized by moderate pain.

54. **Neoplastic disease of the external ear:**
    a. Exostoses are the commonest benign tumours of the cartilage.
    b. Ceruminomas are easily cured by simple excision.
    c. Squamous carcinoma may be associated with xeroderma pigmentosa.
    d. Basal cell carcinomas are usually seen in the external meatus.
    e. An osteoma is composed of ivory bone.

52. *Synopsis 91–92; Scott-Brown 3/6/16–17*
   a. False The causative agent is usually *Pseudomonas aeruginosa*, although *Bacteroides* spp. have also been implicated.
   b. True Extension occurs via the fissures of Santorini, which are natural clefts in the cartilaginous meatus.
   c. False The eardrum is usually intact. The discharge arises from infection and granulations in the external meatus.
   d. True Over 90 per cent of patients are diabetics. Malnutrition, immunosuppression and extremes of age are other important aetiological factors.
   e. True This is due to involvement of the Vth and VIth cranial nerves at the petrous apex. However, VII is the most commonly affected and is a bad prognostic sign. IX, X, XI and XII may be affected.

53. *Synopsis 91; Scott-Brown 3/6/15*
   a. True This is particularly so with herpes zoster, and may involve both the VIIth and XIIth nerves.
   b. True.
   c. True They may precede the rash, usually by several days. The oropharyngeal symptoms are due to vesicles in the buccal mucosa and hard palate.
   d. False It is not effective against the herpes virus harbouring in dorsal root ganglia. Systemic and topical preparations only shorten the period of symptoms.
   e. False The pain is usually excruciating, but settles quite rapidly.

54. *Synopsis 93–95; Scott-Brown 3/6/17–18, 3/22/1–6*
   a. False The origin is the bony canal. The sessile variety is related to cold water (as seen in keen swimmers).
   b. False Wide excision is required due to the frequency of local recurrence. They may progress to adenocarcinomas.
   c. True This is an inherited defect of an enzyme involved in repairing defective DNA.
   d. False They are most common on the auricle.
   e. False It consists of cancellous or spongy bone. Osteomas are usually solitary and pedunculated. Exostoses are of ivory bone, multiple and sessile.

55. **In the external auditory meatus:**
    a. Ceruminous and pilosebaceous glands are located in the cartilaginous meatus.
    b. Keratosis obturans may be associated with bronchiectasis and sinusitis.
    c. Chronic otitis externa may produce a fibrous stenosis.
    d. Vegetable foreign bodies should be syringed with saline.
    e. Live insects may be killed by instillation of oil or spirit.

56. **Congenital anomalies of the middle ear cleft:**
    a. Due to their common origin, the outer, middle and inner ear elements are all affected.
    b. Congenital conductive deafness, with a normal meatus and eardrum, is easily corrected by middle ear microsurgery.
    c. The Treacher-Collins syndrome (mandibulofacial dysostosis) is an autosomal recessive condition associated with major malformations of the outer and middle ear.
    d. In unilateral deformities, middle ear reconstructive surgery is the treatment of choice.
    e. Wildervanck syndrome is a conductive deafness associated with preauricular sinuses and appendages and auricular malformations.

57. **Surgery of congenital ear anomalies:**
    a. A high-resolution CT scan can usually determine which ossicles are present, but rarely shows the exact pathological state.
    b. The facial nerve takes an abnormal course in about 30 per cent of cases, and the fallopian canal is dehiscent in 6 per cent.
    c. A persistent stapedial artery, if present, usually crosses the posterior stapes footplate.
    d. Fusion of the malleus with the incus is one of the commoner abnormalities.
    e. An identifiable tragus is usually associated with a partially-formed external meatus.

55. *Synopsis 83, 95–97; Scott-Brown 1/1/12–14, 3/5/11–12*
    a. True Hair follicles are also situated here.
    b. True It occurs in the younger age group, and appears as a cholesteatomatous mass in the deep meatus.
    c. True.
    d. False Saline will cause them to swell. Surgical spirit should be employed, or patients referred for microscopic suction clearance.
    e. True Only a small amount should be used, otherwise a caloric effect may be produced.

56. *Synopsis 98–100; Scott-Brown 1/1/1–11, 3/4/12, 6/3/9, 6/9/6–12*
    a. False The outer and middle ears are derived from elements of the first and second branchial arches, and the inner ear from the primordial otocyst. Anomalies may occur independently in the two groups.
    b. False Usually the stapes and oval window are affected. The cochlea appears more fragile in these cases, and surgery is therefore hazardous. If deafness has been present since early childhood, it is often misdiagnosed as otosclerosis.
    c. False The condition is autosomal dominant. Facial defects include hypoplastic malar bones, maxillae and mandible.
    d. False No treatment is necessary in most unilateral cases. The bone anchored hearing aid (BAHA), involving a titanium screw implanted into the skull, is safer and more effective than attempts at reconstructive surgery where hearing loss is a problem.
    e. True.

57. *Synopsis 98–100; Scott-Brown 1/1/1–11, 6/3/9, 6/9/6–12*
    a. True.
    b. True. A foreshortened trunk may rise superficial to the posterior annulus; if inferiorly displaced it runs across the promontory. Rarely, the main trunk may be bifid.
    c. False It usually crosses the anterior stapes footplate.
    d. True This forms a single ossicular mass.
    e. True There is therefore a greater chance of surgical success.

58. **Surgical correction of congenital atresia of the external auditory meatus:**
    a. Cases of unilateral atresia do not require investigation.
    b. Exploration in bilateral cases can be deferred until the patient is about 4 years of age.
    c. Plastic reconstruction of the auricle is relatively easy.
    d. Restenosis of a reconstructed external canal is a frequent problem.
    e. External ear remnants are good indicators of the location of the middle ear.

59. **Traumatic perforation of the tympanic membrane:**
    a. Blast rupture affects the pars flaccida.
    b. Tinnitus and vertigo are permanent symptoms.
    c. Blood clot should be syringed out immediately.
    d. Myringoplasty should be performed as early as possible, and always within the first 3 weeks.
    e. Severe pain, requiring analgesia, continues for several days.

60. **In basal skull fractures involving the petrous temporal bone:**
    a. Longitudinal fractures are commoner than transverse, and usually cause conductive deafness.
    b. Transverse fractures commonly cause facial paralysis.
    c. Haemotympanum may present as a blue or black eardrum.
    d. Ecchymosis over the mastoid area may be present.
    e. Sensorineural deafness is usually irreversible.

58. *Synopsis 81–82; Scott-Brown 6/9/1–12*
    a. False It is imperative to check that hearing in the unaffected
            ear is normal. If it is not, rehabilitation must be
            instituted as soon as possible.
    b. True Some advocate a bone-conducting aid until 4–5 years
            of age, followed by surgical correction. Others argue
            that early correction, as young as 2 years, will allow
            better aiding and greater benefit for the acquisition of
            speech.
    c. False This may require several staged operations. A
            prosthesis fitted with titanium bone screws is superior
            to any result achieved with plastic surgery.
    d. True It may be associated with chronic infection. No single
            technique entirely prevents this complication.
    e. False These are not to be relied upon.

59. *Synopsis 100–101; Scott-Brown 1/7/6–10, 3/7/1–3*
    a. False It always affects the pars tensa.
    b. False These are usually transient.
    c. False Never syringe in these cases.
    d. False Many perforations will heal spontaneously. A
            minimum of 6 weeks should be allowed before
            intervening surgically.
    e. False Pain is severe at the time of rupture, but settles very
            rapidly thereafter. Persistent pain implies secondary
            infection.

60. *Synopsis 101–103; Scott-Brown 3/2/13, 3/7/4–8*
    a. True Usually caused by temporal or parietal blows, the
            fracture line runs along the roof of the external
            auditory meatus and middle ear.
    b. True The fracture line involves the labyrinth and internal
            auditory canal. Immediate and complete paralysis has a
            poor prognosis for recovery, and may be an indication
            for urgent exploration via a middle cranial fossa
            approach.
    c. True.
    d. True This is due to bleeding into mastoid air cells
            (Battle's sign).
    e. True It is usually seen in cases of transverse fractures.

61. **Otitic barotrauma:**
    a. In flying, this commonly occurs during descent; in diving, during ascent.
    b. Locking of the Eustachian tube with inability to equilibrate middle ear pressure occurs at a critical pressure difference of about 80 mmHg.
    c. The initial symptoms of ear fullness or blockage are followed by pain and deafness.
    d. This is more likely to occur in cases of mechanical obstruction in the nose.
    e. Resistant cases may require grommet insertion.

62. **Acute suppurative otitis media:**
    a. The degree of mastoid pneumatization influences the clinical picture.
    b. Nasopharyngeal tumours are a very common aetiological factor.
    c. A subperiosteal abscess indicates infective spread beyond the bony cortex.
    d. Tenderness over the mastoid antrum is an important sign elicited by pressure applied in the postauricular sulcus.
    e. Antibiotics are essential if there is to be any hope of resolution.

61. *Synopsis 104–106; Scott-Brown 1/7/1–12*
   a. False It is commoner during descent, both in flying and diving, i.e. when environmental pressure rises above middle ear pressure. Similar damage can occur in compression chambers, and during hyperbaric radiotherapy.
   b. True At this pressure level, the active muscular contraction is not able to open the Eustachian tube.
   c. True.
   d. True Such obstructions include polyps, acute rhinitis, allergic rhinitis or simply a deviated septum.
   e. True Preventive measures include correction of nasal pathology, use of nasal vasoconstrictors, the Valsalva manoeuvre, and chewing sweets prior to and during descents.

62. *Synopsis 106–112; Scott-Brown 3/9/1–10, 6/8/1–5*
   a. True In high degrees of pneumatization a severe clinical course ensues, due to the large mucosal surface area involved in the inflammation.
   b. False Although these can occur in neoplasia of this site, acute rhinitis remains the most common precursor. Any process with the propensity for causing Eustachian salpingitis can be implicated (e.g. sinusitis, nasopharyngitis).
   c. True This will occur more rapidly in a child, due to the thinness of the bony cortex.
   d. False It is elicited by palpation of MacEwen's triangle through the concha.
   e. False The use of antibiotics in uncomplicated acute otitis media is controversial, as most cases will resolve without. If used, they should be appropriate to the infective organism and given in sufficient dosage and continued long enough to ensure complete resolution. Myringotomy is only rarely required. Nasal vaso-constrictors help reduce tubal congestion, but have not been shown to influence outcome in controlled trials.

63. **Acute petrositis:**
    a. This may form a parapharyngeal abscess.
    b. It is a cause of Gradenigo's syndrome.
    c. Simple mastoidectomy may be sufficient treatment, if combined with intravenous antibiotics.
    d. It is of insidious onset, and rarely causes pain or fever.
    e. It can only occur in the 30 per cent of petrous temporal bones that have air cells extending to the apex.

64. **Complications of acute inflammation of the middle ear cleft include the following:**
    a. Febrile convulsions.
    b. Permanent high tone sensorineural hearing loss.
    c. Persistent eardrum perforations.
    d. Acute mastoiditis.
    e. Facial paralysis.

65. **Factors in the development and behaviour of chronic otitis media include the following:**
    a. Bone reaction including erosion and necrosis.
    b. Disorder of middle ear ventilation.
    c. Secondary bacterial infection.
    d. Reactions of the mucoperiosteal lining.
    e. Infiltration by keratinizing stratified squamous epithelium.

63. *Synopsis 110; Scott-Brown 3/9/10, 3/12/5*
  a. True This may occur if the infection coalesces to form a petrous apex abscess, which can tract caudally along the internal carotid artery.
  b. True This is a triad of otorrhoea (continuing mastoid infection), diplopia (VIth cranial nerve involvement) and facial pain (irritation of the Vth cranial nerve).
  c. True If this fails, classic approaches to the petrous apex described by Ramadier, Frenckner and Eagleton may be required. The principle is to follow fistulous tracts to the petrous apex to provide drainage.
  d. False It nearly always occurs in association with either acute otitis media or mastoiditis. A pure infection with Type III pneumococcus has this clinical picture, and may present with an intracranial complication such as meningitis.
  e. True.

64. *Synopsis 110–112; Scott-Brown 3/9/6–10, 6/8/4–5*
  a. True This is especially so in infancy.
  b. True Pus may enter the cochlea via the round or oval window, or may spread via the cochlear aqueduct in cases of otogenic meningitis. The basal turn of the cochlea is first to be affected, but profound deafness at all frequencies can occur if infection spreads to the apex.
  c. True.
  d. True. Bony necrosis of the bony septa of the mastoid air cell system, which coalesce, may occur.
  e. True This occurs in cases of dehiscent facial nerve canals, but normally recovers as the acute infection is controlled either with antibiotic therapy or surgery (myringotomy, cortical mastoidectomy).

65. *Synopsis 112–117; Scott-Brown 3/3/15–30, 3/10/1–2, 3/12/1–2*
  a. True This occurs especially in attico-antral (cholesteatomatous) disease.
  b. True This is particularly so in non-suppurative otitis media (secretory otitis media).
  c. True.
  d. True This occurs especially in tubotympanic CSOM, where there is an increase in the columnar secreting (goblet) cells.
  e. True This occurs in attico-antral (cholesteatomatous) CSOM.

66. **In tubotympanic chronic suppurative otitis media (without cholesteatoma):**
    a. A non-marginal perforation of the pars tensa is usually present.
    b. Erosion of ossicles does not occur unless cholesteatoma develops.
    c. Cholesterol granuloma may occur.
    d. Polypoidal middle ear mucosa and copious mucoid discharge are characteristic.
    e. Intracranial complications will not occur.

67. **Pathogenesis of cholesteatoma:**
    a. Congenital epidermoid rests may break through the outer attic wall.
    b. Squamous epithelium from the external meatus can migrate through a marginal perforation.
    c. Tumarkin's theory postulates an intratympanic negative middle ear pressure with collapse of the eardrum.
    d. Prolonged infection of the middle ear cleft may lead to squamous metaplasia.
    e. Bone erosion is mainly due to a pressure effect.

68. **Clinical features of attico-antral CSOM (with cholesteatoma):**
    a. Deafness is always marked if ossicular damage has occurred.
    b. Copious malodorous otorrhoea is common.
    c. Otalgia is commonly a presenting symptom.
    d. A central perforation is characteristic.
    e. Vertigo is due to blockage of the Eustachian tube.

66. *Synopsis 112–113; Scott-Brown 3/3/15–28, 3/10/1–2, 6/8/5–9*
  a. True The hearing loss is greater if the perforation is posteriorly placed (round window unprotected) rather than anteriorly.
  b. False Erosion of ossicles may occur in all types of CSOM, and results in conductive hearing loss.
  c. True This consists of cholesterol crystals, haemosiderin and other blood pigments, and is one cause of a blue eardrum.
  d. True Discharge is particularly profuse during upper respiratory tract infections.
  e. False Intracranial complications may occur in active chronic otitis media, with or without cholesteatoma.

67. *Synopsis 113–117; Scott-Brown 3/3/18–21, 3/10/1–9, 6/8/14–17*
  a. True Although a possibility, this is considered to be extremely rare. The rests may be activated by an infective episode.
  b. True This is the immigration theory.
  c. True Invagination of the pars flaccida with accumulation of keratin, which enters the attico-antral area after secondary bacterial infection, activates it.
  d. True.
  e. False Enzymatic factors and osteolytic products of chronic infection are the major causes.

68. *Synopsis 113–119; Scott-Brown 3/3/15–30, 3/10/1–9, 3/12/22–27, 6/8/14–19*
  a. False There may be a large conductive loss, but the disease may bridge an ossicular gap, giving near normal hearing.
  b. False This is usually scanty. The offensive odour is due to the decomposing squamous epithelium and, sometimes, osteitis with secondary infection.
  c. False Hearing loss and otorrhoea are the usual symptoms. Earache suggests a complication.
  d. False The perforation is usually marginal, but disease can occur behind an intact eardrum.
  e. False This indicates perilabyrinthitis and potential spread to the inner ear, usually by fistularization of the lateral semicircular canal and, rarely, the promontory.

69. **Management of attico-antral CSOM (with cholesteatoma):**
    a. Intact canal wall mastoidectomy gives excellent access to the sinus tympani.
    b. A posterior tympanotomy provides access to the mesotympanum and hypotympanum by dissection of the facial recess.
    c. Combined approach tympanoplasty is the operation of choice where follow-up cannot be guaranteed.
    d. A type III tympanoplasty (myringostapediopexy) may leave a residual hearing loss of about 25 dB.
    e. No ossicles are sacrificed in a modified radical mastoidectomy.

70. **Management of cholesteatoma in children is difficult for the following reasons:**
    a. Aural toilet may not be tolerated.
    b. Primary epithelialization of mastoid cavities is usual.
    c. There is a high frequency of nasopharyngeal infection.
    d. Excessive fibrosis causes narrowing of the meatoplasty.
    e. There is a high incidence of recurrence with combined approach tympanoplasty.

71. **The discharging mastoid cavity:**
    a. An inadequate meatoplasty, a large cavity, an open tube and the presence of residual disease are all unfavourable factors in these cases.
    b. The Palva flap is an axial pattern vascularized temporalis fascia flap used to line the cavity.
    c. Obliteration with bone paté can be a useful treatment option.
    d. Complete eradication of cholesteatoma is not necessary if a pedicled muscle flap is used to obliterate the cavity.
    e. Only about 40 per cent heal satisfactorily.

69. *Synopsis 35, 113–117; Scott-Brown 1/1/19, 3/10/6–8, 3/11/1–8, 6/8/14–19*
- a. False With this approach, there is a high risk of leaving cholesteatoma in this site. An atticotomy/antrostomy approach is little better, and the sinus tympani is the commonest site of residual cholesteatoma with all forms of mastoidectomy. Intraoperative use of the Storz-Hopkins teleotoscope may improve visualization of the sinus tympani.
- b. True.
- c. False There is a very high recurrence rate. Most will require a 'second look' operation, and ultimately may need a wide access procedure.
- d. True.
- e. False The incus and malleus head are removed.

70. *Synopsis 113–115; Scott-Brown 6/8/5–21*
- a. True.
- b. False Children produce excessive fibrogranular tissue, leading to chronically discharging cavities.
- c. True This is especially so up to the age of 11 years. Adenoidectomy, tonsillectomy and attention to maxillary sinuses may be indicated.
- d. True This is due to an exuberant healing process.
- e. True The risk of recurrent cholesteatoma is so high with closed techniques that exteriorization, despite the drawbacks above, is preferred by many surgeons.

71. *Synopsis 35, 113–117; Scott-Brown 3/3/30–33, 3/10/6–8, 3/11/1–7, 6/8/5–21*
- a. True.
- b. False The Palva flap is a random pattern muscle flap.
- c. True All active infection should be eradicated from the site.
- d. False It is essential to eradicate all disease.
- e. False This figure is nearer 70–80 per cent in experienced hands.

72. **Acute mastoiditis:**
    a. This is most common in young children.
    b. A postauricular swelling with anterior displacement of the pinna is the commonest presenting sign.
    c. Sagging of the posterosuperior meatal wall is an important diagnostic sign.
    d. Parenteral antibiotics should be given only after confirmation of the infecting organism by culture and sensitivity.
    e. Surgery, normally a simple cortical mastoidectomy, is necessary if a subperiosteal abscess has formed.

73. **Intracranial extension of suppurative otitis media:**
    a. This can occur due to bone erosion by cholesteatoma.
    b. Extension may be through the petrosquamous suture line.
    c. It may extend, via the labyrinth, along the aqueduct of the cochlea.
    d. Extension through the mastoid emissary vein is possible.
    e. Extension along a dehiscent facial canal is rare.

72. *Synopsis 108–110; Scott-Brown 3/9/7–10, 6/8/4–5*
    a. True   Up to 40 per cent occur in children under 1 year old.
    b. True   However, this is not always present.
    c. True   This is frequently associated with a perforation and pus from the middle ear.
    d. False Broad-spectrum intravenous antibiotics should be commenced immediately. Common infective organisms are beta-haemolytic streptococcus and type III pneumococcus. Anaerobes may also be present, and should be covered in the chosen antibiotic regimen. Pus for culture may be obtained from the meatus if the drum has perforated, from a myringotomy, or from the abscess itself when it is drained.
    e. True   It is usually sufficient simply to 'uncap' the mastoid cortex. A myringotomy is necessary if the drum has not already perforated. An attempt to exenterate all mastoid air cells in the presence of active infection and bleeding granulations risks damage to the facial nerve.

73. *Synopsis 117–119; Scott-Brown 1/1/20–27, 3/3/18–25, 3/12/1–27, 6/8/4–5*
    a. True   This explains the old distinction between 'safe' (tubo-tympanic) and 'unsafe' (attico-antral, cholesteatoma) CSOM. This myth was conclusively disproved by Browning in his study of the neurosurgical complications of both types of CSOM in the West of Scotland.
    b. True   This may occur if the suture line is non-united. It occurs less frequently through the squamomastoid or occipitomastoid sutures.
    c. True   Once in the labyrinth, there are also preformed pathways along the internal auditory canal and the vestibular aqueduct.
    d. True   Extension may also occur via vascular foraminae in MacEwan's triangle.
    e. True   However, this is certainly possible.

74. **Complications of suppurative otitis media:**
    a. These include a retropharyngeal abscess.
    b. They rarely involve the middle cranial fossa because of the resistance of the tegmen antri and tympani.
    c. Complications may give a positive Tobey-Ayer test.
    d. They are more likely to give rise to otogenic intracranial hypertension with the left ear.
    e. Complications may be confused with mumps.

75. **Otitis media with effusion (secretory otitis media, SOM):**
    a. Is most prevalent in the second decade of life.
    b. Eustachian tube dysfunction is an important aetiological factor.
    c. This is more likely in the presence of large infected adenoids.
    d. Passive smoking is the major cause in the developed world.
    e. Bacterial infection is unlikely to play any role, because the effusion is sterile.

The ear

74. *Synopsis 117–119; Scott-Brown 3/12/1–27, 6/8/4–5*
  a. True   A parapharyngeal abscess is also possible, as pus can track along peritubal cells.
  b. False   Both are frequent sites of extension of disease.
  c. True   In cases of occluding thrombus in the lateral venous sinus, no rise in CSF on manometry is noted on ipsilateral internal jugular vein compression. It is a late sign.
  d. False   The superior sagittal sinus more frequently drains into the right lateral sinus. Retrograde thrombophlebitis blocking the arachnoid villi in the former sinus is the pathophysiological basis of otitic hydrocephalus.
  e. True   A zygomatic abscess may form deep to the temporalis muscle, mimicking a parotitis.

75. *Synopsis 119–122; Scott-Brown 6/7/1–6*
  a. False   It is most prevalent in the first decade. Older studies indicated a peak prevalence around the age of 4–6 years, but this was probably a reflection of the population studied and the diagnostic criteria employed. It is now believed that the peak prevalence may be in those under 2 years of age.
  b. True   Before the age of 5 years, the normal tube is shorter and lies in a horizontal plane. This position detracts from the efficiency of the muscles responsible for opening it. However, in cleft palate cases, additional anatomical defects of the Eustachian tube account for the high prevalence of SOM.
  c. True   Not due to physical blockage of the Eustachian tube by the mass of adenoids, but probably reduced tubal patency consequent upon an ascending salpingitis.
  d. False   Studies have given conflicting results. Passive smoking does play a role, but is not the major cause.
  e. False   Pathogenic bacteria can be cultured in around 30 per cent of cases.

76. **Diagnosis and management of otitis media with effusion:**
    a. Varying the head posture may alter the degree of deafness.
    b. Pain is an uncommon feature.
    c. A mobile eardrum excludes the diagnosis.
    d. Cortical mastoidectomy may be necessary.
    e. Grommet insertion is ineffective and unnecessary.

77. **Late sequelae of otitis media with effusion:**
    a. Middle ear atelectasis is related to the overall duration and severity of the disease.
    b. Adhesive otitis media can be satisfactorily managed by division of fibrous bands and insertion of silastic sheeting.
    c. An attic retraction pocket may form the basis for cholesteatoma formation, and can be reliably prevented by grommet insertion.
    d. Tympanosclerosis is commoner in ears that have been treated by grommet insertion.
    e. The use of long-term ventilation tubes is associated with a high risk of perforation (around 20 per cent).

78. **Tuberculous otitis media has the following characteristics:**
    a. It is usually painless.
    b. It is associated with multiple perforations of the pars tensa.
    c. It is occasionally heralded by a mastoid complication such as facial paralysis.
    d. It is possibly contracted by aspiration of milk via the Eustachian tube.
    e. It is caused by *Treponema pallidum*.

76. *Synopsis 119–122; Scott-Brown 6/7/6–17*
  a. True   This is particularly so if the middle ear fluid is thin. Hearing is best in bed.
  b. True   This is more likely to occur in an acute secretory otitis media caused by flying or diving with an upper respiratory tract infection.
  c. False Although mobility is usually absent, an early or resolving effusion may have a mobile eardrum.
  d. True   Cases resistant to conventional treatment may have a coexisting secretory mastoiditis.
  e. False Grommet insertion gives immediate relief from the disability of hearing loss. It should be reserved for more severe cases, which show no tendency to spontaneous resolution.

77. *Synopsis 122–123; Scott-Brown 6/7/14–17*
  a. True.
  b. False Surgery is usually fruitless, due to the recurrent formation of adhesions and the risk of sensorineural deafness with ossicular reconstruction. The provision of a hearing aid is frequently the best management.
  c. False The attic retraction pocket may develop into a cholesteatoma, but insertion of grommets does not necessarily prevent this from occurring.
  d. True   However, tympanosclerosis confined to the drum has no significant adverse effect on hearing.
  e. True.

78. *Synopsis 123–124; Scott-Brown 1/19/12–13, 3/2/16, 3/3/18, 3/10/8, 3/15/29–30*
  a. True.
  b. True   These may eventually coalesce to produce a single large defect. Pale granulations are frequently present.
  c. True   There may also be a cold subperiosteal abscess, labyrinthine fistula and tuberculous meningitis (particularly in young patients).
  d. True   This occurred with cow's milk infected by bovine tuberculosis in prepasteurization days. Infection secondary to pulmonary tuberculosis, or with atypical mycobacteria in AIDS, is the usual cause nowadays.
  e. False It is caused by *Mycobacterium tuberculosis*. The treponeme is the infective organism of syphilis.

79. **Malignant tumours of the middle ear cleft:**
    a. Adenocarcimona is the commonest histological type.
    b. Squamous carcinoma is usually associated with chronic otitis media.
    c. Intense pain is caused by meningeal involvement.
    d. Adenocarcinoma is radiosensitive and so surgery is reserved for residual or recurrent disease.
    e. Radical mastoidectomy is usually performed prior to radiotherapy.

80. **Paragangliomas of the temporal bone:**
    a. These are more aggressive histologically than glomus tumours.
    b. They may present with involvement of the IXth, Xth and XIth cranial nerves.
    c. They are more common in males.
    d. Because they are benign, radiotherapy plays no part in their management.
    e. They may occur concurrently with a carotid body tumour.

81. **Osseous disorders of the temporal bone:**
    a. Monostotic fibrous dysplasia is more common than the polyostotic type.
    b. Paget's disease (osteitis deformans) characteristically causes a progressive mixed conductive and sensorineural hearing loss.
    c. Eosinophilic granuloma produces punched out lesions, which are seen on plain X-rays.
    d. Osteopetrosis (marble bone disease) may cause blindness, conductive hearing loss and recurrent facial palsies.
    e. The eosinophilic granuloma type of histiocytosis-X may present as a painful mastoid swelling with a solitary osteolytic lesion.

79. *Synopsis 127–128; Scott-Brown 3/22/1–6*
 a. False Squamous carcinoma is commonest. Adenocarcinoma is very rare, and is usually due to direct extension of an adenocarcinoma of the external canal or deep lobe of the parotid.
 b. True Chronic otorrhoea probably causes squamous metaplasia. There is usually a very long history of CSOM. Many cases occur in chronically infected mastoidectomy cavities.
 c. True Pain, either its appearance or increase, is a suspicious symptom in a chronic suppurative otitis media.
 d. False Adenocarcinoma is radioresistant. Radical surgery offers the only hope of a cure.
 e. True This allows an appreciation of the extent of disease, drainage, relief of pain and sepsis. The cavity can be more easily reviewed post-operatively and post-irradiation.

80. *Synopsis 125; Scott-Brown 3/23/1–16*
 a. False The terms are synonymous. Aggressiveness refers to the clinical behaviour of a tumour rather than its histology.
 b. True This is the so-called 'jugular foramen syndrome', which may occur in glomus jugulare tumours.
 c. False Over 70 per cent of these cases are female.
 d. False They are of low grade malignancy, and can occasionally metastasize. Radiotherapy is a useful adjunct to surgical resection. In patients with massive intracranial extension, or elderly patients unfit for surgery, radiotherapy can prevent progression for several years.
 e. True Paraganglionic tissue is also found in the turbinates, vagal bodies, larynx and aorta. All can give rise to paragangliomas.

81. *Synopsis 133–135; Scott-Brown 3/4/36–46, 3/15/1–44*
 a. True Hyperparathyroidism should be excluded. Radiotherapy should be avoided, as it predisposes to malignant change.
 b. True This is due to the involvement of the malleus and incus, cochlea, and internal auditory canal. The stapes footplate is rarely affected.
 c. True Conductive loss is due to ossicular involvement.
 d. True This is due to involvement of cranial nerve foramina in the skull base.
 e. True.

82. **Pathology of otosclerosis:**
    a. Mature lamellar bone is removed and replaced by spongy osteoid bone.
    b. The commonest site for the otosclerotic lesion is in the posterior promontory in the region of the fossula post-fenestram.
    c. Blue mantles of Manasse are due to venous congestion in the active focus, and can be seen clearly under high magnification of the operating microscope.
    d. About 80 per cent of cases are bilateral.
    e. Possible causes of cochlear otosclerosis include bone deposition in the scala tympani, impaired microcirculation of the stria vascularis by adjacent active foci, and damage to the organ of Corti by toxic metabolites.

83. **Patients with otosclerosis:**
    a. Patients are commonly of black African race.
    b. They may notice an onset or increase of deafness during pregnancy.
    c. Patients without a family history may represent new mutations.
    d. There is a female to male ratio of 2:1.
    e. In 70 per cent of cases, they first show symptoms between 45 and 55 years of age.

84. **Diagnosis of otosclerosis:**
    a. Paracusis Willisi may be present.
    b. Carhart's notches at 500 and 1000 Hz are seen on pure tone audiometric thresholds with air conduction.
    c. Tympanometry is of little value.
    d. Vertigo is usually due to a labyrinthine hydrops.
    e. Differential diagnosis from congenital footplate fixation is difficult, as the conductive hearing loss is also progressive.

82. *Synopsis 129–133; Scott-Brown 3/4/45–46, 3/14/2–5, 3/15/3–8*
    a. True The latter is of greater thickness, cellularity and vascularity; hence the more apt descriptive term 'otospongiosis', used by Europeans.
    b. False 85 per cent of cases occur anterior to the oval window in the fissula ante-fenestram. This is a site of unossified bone.
    c. False The blue mantles of Manasse are histological features of the active focus, seen with haematoxylin and eosin staining.
    d. True.
    e. True.

83. *Synopsis 129–133; Scott-Brown 3/14/2–7*
    a. False Most patients are Caucasian.
    b. True This is particularly so about term. Thyrotoxicosis or onset of the menopause may also increase otosclerotic deafness. It is probably related to the hormonal milieu and high metabolic activity.
    c. True However, isolated cases may be a misdiagnosis, or relatives may have histological otosclerosis without hearing loss.
    d. True.
    e. False 90 per cent of the cases seen are aged 15–45 years, peaking in the third decade.

84. *Synopsis 129–133; Scott-Brown 3/14/2–11*
    a. True This is the phenomenon of hearing better in a background of noise.
    b. False Notches are seen on bone conduction. Carhart's notch at 2000 Hz is most common, although other notches occur.
    c. False It can differentiate middle ear pathologies that mimic otosclerosis (ossicular discontinuity, fixed malleus/incus, etc.); the measure of compliance gives an indication as to the type of footplate likely to be encountered during surgery.
    d. False This is probably due to the toxic effects of enzymes liberated by the otosclerotic focus on the vestibular labyrinth. The commonest clinical type is benign positional vertigo. Hydrops may occur, but it is rare.
    e. False In congenital footplate fixation, the hearing loss is frequently noted from early childhood and is non-progressive.

85. **Treatment of otosclerosis:**
    a. Sodium fluoride therapy is employed in cochlear otosclerosis.
    b. Hearing aids halt the progression of otosclerosis.
    c. Surgery is of less benefit to the patient with a normal contralateral ear than to bilateral cases.
    d. Sensorineural losses may occur as late as 10 years after initially successful stapedectomy.
    e. Fluorides may be administered safely during pregnancy.

86. **During stapes surgery:**
    a. Perilymph flooding may be due to an abnormally patent cochlear aqueduct.
    b. Total removal of the footplate is safer than drilling a small fenestra, because the hydraulic effect on the membranous labyrinth is less.
    c. The facial nerve presents no problems if it is in an intact fallopian canal.
    d. Blood or bone chips in the vestibule should be sucked out immediately to prevent toxic effects on the labyrinth.
    e. A persistent stapedial artery is encountered in about 3 per cent of stapes surgery cases.

85. *Synopsis 129–133; Scott-Brown 3/14/11–31, 3/15/6*
  a. True Its use is not universally accepted by otologists.
  b. False This is utter nonsense. Hearing aids provide amplification. Aids with or without tinnitus maskers may be indicated.
  c. True The potential benefit of surgery is less where the contralateral ear is normal. Successful surgery in a unilateral case does, however, allow the bonus of binaural hearing and sound localization.
  d. True Losses are more likely to occur with large fenestra or total removal of the footplate, and less likely with a small fenestra and vein graft.
  e. False.

86. *Synopsis 129–133; Scott-Brown 3/14/15–31*
  a. True This is an unusual complication, commoner in congenital stapes fixation than in otosclerosis. It may be possible to control by raising the head, administering parenteral mannitol or inserting a spinal drain.
  b. False The opposite is true.
  c. False The canal itself may bulge down, obscuring the oval window.
  d. False Bleeding into the vestibule should be avoided by having a dry field. If it does occur, suction should be avoided, because the definite risk of mechanical trauma outweighs any theoretical risk of toxic effects. Bone chips should not occur in the small fenestra drilling technique. If they occur in stapedectomy, they should be removed gently with a fine hook or pick, not with suction.
  e. False This is encountered in about 0.3 per cent of cases.

87. **Complications of stapedectomy:**
   a. A divided chorda tympani always produces a loss or alteration of taste.
   b. Balance disturbance in the early post-operative period should be treated by vestibular exercises.
   c. Conductive hearing loss may be due to incus dislocation.
   d. An over-long piston is better than one that is short.
   e. Incus tip necrosis is the most frequent cause of recurrent conductive deafness.

88. **Perilymph fistulae following stapedectomy:**
   a. A primary fistula is due to failure to achieve an adequate seal of the opening into the vestibule around the prosthesis at operation.
   b. A secondary fistula may be submucosal and track up the shaft of the prosthesis.
   c. Fluctuating hearing loss is a cardinal sign of a large fistula.
   d. Tinnitus and hearing loss are usually improved if closure is successful.
   e. The Fraser test may be positive.

87. *Synopsis 129–133; Scott-Brown 3/14/18–31*
   a. False There may be no subjective complaints.
   b. False All strain and sudden head movements should be
             avoided, particularly straining during defecation.
             Flying, travelling by underground train or travel over
             high mountain passes should be avoided for 2 weeks.
             Sneezing with the nose and/or mouth closed should
             also be avoided. Vestibular exercises may be helpful
             later in cases of labyrinthine damage, by hastening
             adaptation.
   c. True.
   d. False The former is worse due to the high risk of early and
             late perilymph fistulae and subsequent sensorineural
             losses. The latter produce only a mechanical failure
             leading to persistent conductive hearing loss.
   e. False A slipped prosthesis is the usual culprit, with a
             conductive hearing loss of about 60 dB and high
             compliance values.

88. *Synopsis 129–133; Scott-Brown 3/14/24–26*
   a. True   Vein grafting combined with small fenestra minimizes
            the risk.
   b. True   Other sites are at the oval window margin, and
            through a defect in the soft tissue graft at the medial
            end of the prosthesis.
   c. False Small fistulae are more likely to exhibit this sign,
            presumably because the leak is intermittent. With a
            large fistula, the loss is likely to be of rapid onset and
            non-fluctuating.
   d. False Vertigo is helped and hearing loss may be improved if
            repair is affected early (usually not the case), but
            tinnitus is rarely ameliorated. The tendency is for the
            diagnosis to be considered too late for effective action.
   e. True   The test is positive if, after 20 minutes with the
            affected ear uppermost, there is an improvement in
            the pure tone and/or speech audiometry. The
            pathophysiological basis is an air bubble in the cochlea
            causing a 'cochlear-conductive' hearing loss.

89. **Van der Hoeve de Kleyn syndrome:**
    a. Microscopic fractures with subsequent healing are the probable cause of stapedovestibular fixation.
    b. Deafness does not occur without evidence of fractures.
    c. Compliance values are low.
    d. Stapedectomy is usually deferred until several years after spontaneous fractures have ceased.
    e. Amelogenesis imperfecta may be associated.

90. **In late syphilis in the temporal bone:**
    a. Cochlear duct hydrops is a common feature.
    b. Hennebert's sign may be positive.
    c. Steroids may improve the hearing deficit.
    d. Interstitial keratitis may have occurred several years previously.
    e. The Tullio phenomenon (transient vertigo and nystagmus induced by sudden loud noise) may occur due to dilatation of the saccule.

89. *Synopsis 133; Scott-Brown 3/4/38–40; 3/15/9–10*
 a. True.
 b. False   Deafness or deafness and blue sclerae can occur without fractures.
 c. False   Values are usually very high, despite ossicular fixation, probably due to abnormal collagen causing excessive laxity of the eardrum.
 d. True   The results are not as successful as in otosclerosis. There is a greater risk of a floating footplate, and the bone may be thick and vascular, causing excessive haemorrhage.
 e. True   This occurs in about 15 per cent of cases. There is irregular dentine formation, with yellow, opaque, irregular teeth.

90. *Synopsis 124, 152–153; Scott-Brown 3/4/25–26, 3/15/25–29*
 a. True   The saccule and utricle are also involved. Sudden total or profound hearing loss may be due to rupture of the cochlear duct.
 b. True   This is a sign of a fistula, with an intact drum and no middle ear disease. Pathophysiologically, it is due to energy transmission via the stapes footplate directly onto a distended saccule.
 c. True   They should be given in combination with an appropriate antitreponemal agent such as benzylpenicillin.
 d. True.
 e. True   Dilatation of the saccule allows sound energy transmission from the stapes footplate. The same pathophysiological mechanism also explains Hennebert's sign.

91. Congenital deafness:
  a. Maternal rubella in the second trimester is a common prenatal cause of sensorineural deafness.
  b. A white forelock and heterochromia iridium may be associated with an autosomal dominant hereditary deafness.
  c. Screening tests can only be reliably performed on patients over 12 months of age.
  d. A high tone loss is characteristic of cases caused by rhesus incompatibility.
  e. Electric response audiometry is not particularly useful in assessing auditory function.

92. Temporal bone fractures:
  a. About 80 per cent are longitudinal, running along the roof of the external meatus and middle ear, then anterior to the bony labyrinth.
  b. Conductive hearing loss is characteristic of longitudinal fractures, and sensorineural hearing loss of transverse fractures.
  c. A late sequel of disequilibrium may be exacerbated by physical fatigue.
  d. Facial paralysis is seen in about 50 per cent of transverse fractures.
  e. The prognosis for recovery of sensorineural hearing loss is better in transverse than in longitudinal fractures.

93. In closed head injuries without fracture:
  a. Hearing loss, if present, is most marked at 4000 Hz.
  b. The most common vestibular symptom is positional vertigo.
  c. Unilateral canal paresis is common.
  d. Latent nystagmus may be revealed by removal of optic fixation.
  e. Rapid acceleration may cause cochlear vestibular damage.

91. *Synopsis 136–141; Scott-Brown 3/4/1–26, 6/3/1–18, 6/4/1–19*
    a. False The virus affects the developing labyrinth in the first trimester. It was a common prenatal cause of deafness, but is becoming less so. A policy of vaccination of all children aims to greatly reduce the pool of infection in the community, and hence cut the incidence of congenital rubella.
    b. True This is Waardenburg syndrome. It also includes the features of a broad nasal bridge and lateral displacement of the medial canthi.
    c. False Tests can and should be conducted as early as possible.
    d. True.
    e. False It can provide very reliable objective measurement of thresholds in very young children, and will allow differentiation from those suffering from multiple neurological deficits (e.g. in cerebral palsy) but whose hearing thresholds are normal.

92. *Synopsis 141–142; Scott-Brown 3/7/4–8*
    a. True.
    b. True However, there may be a mixed picture with either type. The conductive loss may be temporary due to haemo-tympanum, or permanent due to ossicular disruption.
    c. True In unilateral vestibular failure, the subsequent compensation may break down if other sources of sensory information are excluded (e.g. due to failing eyesight, fatigue, illness and drugs).
    d. True.
    e. False A transverse fracture usually passes through the vestibule and is associated with severe or total sensorineural hearing loss, which will not recover. The high tone loss that often accompanies a longitudinal fracture may well recover.

93. *Synopsis 142–3; Scott-Brown 3/7/4–9*
    a. True It is usually bilateral.
    b. True This is of the benign paroxysmal variety. Perilymph fistulae, due to labyrinthine membrane rupture, may also be present.
    c. True This occurs in about 60 per cent of ears.
    d. True.
    e. True This is due to the relative inertia of the brain in relation to the skull.

94. **Inner ear barotrauma:**
    a. A Valsalva manoeuvre during a deep sea dive, in the presence of a locked Eustachian tube, may cause labyrinthine window rupture.
    b. Decompression sickness is best treated by giving an oxygen–helium breathing mixture.
    c. Patients with a short, wide cochlear aqueduct are more prone to problems.
    d. A previous stapedectomy reduces the risk of damage during flying.
    e. Unilateral labyrinthine failure can be caused by changing from an oxyhelium gas mix to compressed air at the start of decompression.

95. **Excessive sound stimulation of the ear:**
    a. This may cause transitory residual masking.
    b. A long-lasting temporary threshold shift (TTS) recovers within 16 hours.
    c. This can produce an acoustic notch at 6000 Hz.
    d. A short, intense single noise exposure may lead to permanent sensorineural deafness.
    e. This can evoke the Tullio phenomenon only with an intact and mobile middle ear mechanism.

96. **Infrasound:**
    a. Infrasound is easily detected by the human ear.
    b. It occurs in high-speed automobiles, particularly if the windows are open.
    c. It may induce nystagmus.
    d. It could have caused the destruction of the Walls of Jericho.
    e. It can be recorded on a normal tape recorder.

94. *Synopsis 104–106, 148; Scott-Brown 1/7/10–16, 3/7/9–10*
   a. True   Any diver with persistent giddiness or sensorineural
             deafness should be suspected of having a labyrinthine
             membrane rupture.
   b. False Recompression is essential. This prevents gas bubbles
             within the inner ear.
   c. True   The infantile aqueduct is only 3.5 mm long and is of
             relatively wide bore. This may persist into adulthood. It
             is unable to smooth out fluctuations in pressure
             differentials between the CSF and perilymph.
   d. False The reverse is true.
   e. True   Gas bubbles are believed to form at the middle ear/
             inner ear interface.

95. *Synopsis 143–147; Scott-Brown 2/11/1–34*
   a. True   Transitory residual masking is a physiological adaptive
             phenomenon. A loud sound (up to 90 dB) elevates the
             threshold for an identical frequency presented
             immediately afterwards. Frequencies above and below
             are affected to a lesser degree. Rapid exponential
             recovery occurs, within 0.5 s for sounds up to 70 dB.
   b. False Long-lasting TTSs are of greater than 16 hours' duration,
             and merge imperceptibly with permanent threshold shifts.
   c. True   However, a 4000 Hz dip is most commonly seen in
             practice. 6000 Hz is not a frequency that is tested on
             routine audiometry, but losses at 3000 or 6000 Hz may
             occur earlier than the classical 4000 Hz dip.
   d. True   This is termed 'acoustic trauma'.
   e. True   This is the term applied to noise-induced vertigo,
             which is probably due to excessive medial displacement
             of the stapes causing contact with a dilated saccule.

96. *Synopsis – no specific reference; Scott-Brown 2/11/20–21*
   a. False By definition, infrasound is below the lower frequency
             limit of hearing. The ear is a very poor detector of
             sounds below 16 Hz.
   b. True   This accounts for some of the unpleasant sensations of
             light-headedness and nausea that may be experienced.
   c. True   This is probably induced by the Tullio phenomenon
             principle.
   d. True   This could be possible if the correct resonant
             frequency had been emitted by the trumpets.
   e. False It requires an FM (frequency modulation) tape recorder.

97. **Hearing conservation programmes in industry:**
    a. A sound profile of the potentially hazardous area is essential.
    b. Temporary threshold shifts do not adversely affect audiometric testing.
    c. The most effective hearing protector is the earmuff.
    d. Hearing protection need not be worn continuously in a high-risk zone.
    e. Observation booths may be a practical solution.

98. **Otitic blast injury:**
    a. The first phase (positive pressure wave) damages the tympanic membrane, while the second phase (negative pressure wave) is more likely to damage the inner ear.
    b. The injury may be complicated by squamous epithelial cysts developing in the middle ear.
    c. The extent of damage to the inner ear is reduced by an accompanying rupture of the eardrum.
    d. This injury only infrequently produces tinnitus.
    e. It does not produce vestibular symptoms.

99. **Labyrinthine window rupture:**
    a. A preceding history of trauma can always be elicited.
    b. The round window is more frequently affected than the oval window.
    c. Symptoms and audiometry may be similar to those of Ménière's disease.
    d. A rupture is usually visualized under high magnification.
    e. Surgical closure improves the hearing in over 60 per cent of cases.

The ear

97. *Synopsis 145–147; Scott-Brown 2/11/25–28*
   a. True   For example, measurements of noise levels at various points should be taken.
   b. False   As the shift may be as high as 30 dB, sufficient time between noise exposure and testing should be allowed to minimize this problem.
   c. True   If properly fitted, they can attenuate up to 50 dB in the higher frequencies.
   d. False   Non-adherence for even as little as a few minutes considerably reduces the value of protective measures.
   e. True   These separate the operative from the sound source.

98. *Synopsis 146; Scott-Brown 2/11/13, 3/7/1–3, 10–11, 3/16/3*
   a. True.
   b. True   These may be from implanted fragments or inversion of the edges of the perforation.
   c. False   Temporary or permanent sensorineural deafness is frequently seen despite the presence of perforations.
   d. False   Tinnitus is an invariable symptom, but usually resolves spontaneously.
   e. False   Benign paroxysmal positional vertigo may be observed. Perilymph fistulae may also occur.

99. *Synopsis 3/7/9–10; Scott-Brown 1/7/11–16, 3/7/9–10, 3/14/24–27*
   a. False   Although trauma is frequent (closed head injury, barotrauma), even slight exertion (lifting, sneezing, coitus) causing a rise in intracranial pressure may be the initiating factor. Spontaneous ruptures may rarely occur.
   b. False   The reverse is true, and occasionally both are involved.
   c. True   In such cases, a positive Fraser's test is highly suggestive of a perilymph leak.
   d. False   Frequently, its presence can only be inferred from the leakage of fluid. Normal seepage of tissue fluid or injected infiltration solution can mislead the surgeon. Jugular pressure, the head-down position and Valsalva under general anaesthetic are manoeuvres that can be employed if there is no obvious leak, but they have the disadvantage that venous oozing may be induced.
   e. False   Hearing is improved in about 30 per cent of cases. Vestibular symptoms are relieved in about 80 per cent of cases. Tinnitus is rarely improved.

100. **Otitic labyrinthitis:**
    a. This is most commonly due to surgical trauma such as stapedectomy or mastoidectomy.
    b. It may be produced by a pathological fistula.
    c. It can occur after an acute viral illness.
    d. It may result in ossification of the auditory nerve.
    e. It cannot occur by direct spread of middle ear infection via the labyrinthine window membranes, since they are impermeable.

101. **In circumscribed labyrinthitis:**
    a. Symptoms may be precipitated by auricular movement.
    b. Auto-inflation is the most effective method of eliciting the fistula sign.
    c. In a weakly positive fistula sign, nystagmus without vertigo is elicited.
    d. If there is no obvious cholesteatoma, long-term conservative management is indicated.
    e. The hearing deficit will not recover.

102. **Effects of AIDS on the ear:**
    a. Otitis media with effusion may occur due to lymphoid hypertrophy in the nasopharynx.
    b. Patients may present with sudden or fluctuating sensorineural deafness.
    c. Labyrinthine cryptococcosis occurs due to opportunistic infection when cell-mediated immunity is impaired.
    d. Kaposi's sarcoma is limited to the skin of the external ear.
    e. The HIV virus may activate latent otosyphilis.

100. *Synopsis 148–152; Scott-Brown 3/3/23, 3/12/22–26*
    a. False   Chronic suppurative otitis media with extension is the commonest aetiological factor.
    b. True   It is usually due to erosion of the lateral semicircular canal or, occasionally, the promontory. If the membranous labyrinth is not breached, this condition may only produce symptoms during the fistula test. Terms employed for this condition include paralabyrinthitis, perilabyrinthitis and circumscribed labyrinthitis.
    c. True   Acute coryza (adenovirus type 3), mumps, measles or herpes zoster may accompany myringitis bullosa haemorrhagica.
    d. False   There may be sclerosis (labyrinthitis ossificans) in both the vestibule and cochlea as the end result of suppurative labyrinthitis.
    e. False   Direct spread can occur in acute infections.

101. *Synopsis 148–152; Scott-Brown 3/3/23, 3/12/22–26*
    a. True   Symptoms may also be precipitated by head movement, sneezing and coughing.
    b. False   Pneumomassage with Siegle's speculum or rhythmical tragal pressure may elicit the nystagmus and vertigo.
    c. False   Nystagmus is absent but vertigo is present.
    d. False   Some form of mastoid exploration will be required. Exteriorization is essential.
    e. False   The deficit may improve.

102. *Synopsis – no specific reference; Scott-Brown 3/3/13, 3/4/26–27, 3/17/7–9*
    a. True   It may also be due to chronic rhino-sinusitis and, rarely, to nasopharyngeal tumours such as Kaposi's sarcoma.
    b. True.
    c. True   This occurs in severe cases, and may form part of the terminal illness.
    d. False   It may affect the middle ear, and has been reported to metastasize to the auditory nerve.
    e. True   Many HIV-positive patients have a past history of syphilis. Reduced cell-mediated immunity accelerates progress to tertiary manifestations.

103. **Pathophysiology of Ménière's disease:**
    a. The negative summating potential on electrocochleography is enhanced due to stretching and stiffening of the basilar membrane.
    b. There is gross dilatation of the scala vestibuli.
    c. Fibrous bands may connect the footplate to the distended saccule.
    d. Ruptures of the membranous labyrinth have been postulated as the cause of acute attacks.
    e. Sodium and potassium levels in the endolymph are grossly abnormal.

104. **Clinical manifestations of Ménière's disease:**
    a. Vertiginous attacks characteristically occur without warning.
    b. Utricular crises are common.
    c. Horizontal nystagmus is absent during an acute crisis.
    d. Migrainous headaches may be associated with vertiginous attacks.
    e. Diplacusis is a suggestive diagnostic feature.

105. **Cogan's syndrome is characterized by the following:**
    a. Audiovestibular symptoms and interstitial keratitis.
    b. Vertigo without hearing loss or tinnitus.
    c. An improvement in hearing and tinnitus with the onset of vertigo.
    d. Copious otorrhoea.
    e. Radiological expansion of the internal auditory canal.

103. *Synopsis 153–158; Scott-Brown 3/1/25, 3/17/30–31, 3/19/4–24*
  a. True   The normal summating potential occurs because
             the basilar membrane becomes displaced towards
             the scala media with high intensity stimulation. In
             endolymphatic hydrops, the membrane is already
             displaced and stretched; hence the summating potential
             is both wider and deeper in Ménière's disease.
  b. False   The scala media (cochlear duct) and saccule are
             dilated.
  c. True.
  d. True   Rupture and subsequent healing may explain the
             exacerbations and remissions that characterize
             Ménière's disease.
  e. False   Most studies show that levels of these cations are
             relatively normal.

104. *Synopsis 153–158; Scott-Brown 3/19/14–18*
  a. False   About 50 per cent of patients have prodromal
             symptoms such as muffled hearing, heaviness or
             pressure in the ear. Some attacks start with
             increasing loudness of tinnitus or a change in its
             character, often described as 'roaring'.
  b. False   These are also known as 'drop attacks', and are
             very uncommon. They occur without warning.
  c. False   It is always present, and its direction may vary
             between and during attacks. Between attacks it may
             be elicited only by ENG with abolition of optic
             fixation.
  d. True   Some claim the association in as many as 20 per
             cent of cases.
  e. True   A sound of a given frequency is perceived to be a
             different pitch in each ear.

105. *Synopsis 161; Scott-Brown 3/4/11, 3/5/14, 3/15/41–42,
        3/17/23–24, 3/19/18*
  a. True   The keratitis is non-syphilitic.
  b. False.
  c. False   These are the symptoms of Lermoyez syndrome, a
             rare variant of Ménière's disease.
  d. False.
  e. False.

106. **Investigation of Ménière's disease:**
   a. A normal caloric response excludes the diagnosis.
   b. The glycerol dehydration test is especially useful in patients with near normal hearing.
   c. Speech audiometry is helpful in differentiation between sensory and neural deafness.
   d. Electrocochleography may reveal changes in the unaffected ear.
   e. Vestibular aqueduct tomography is essential.

107. **Medical management of Ménière's disease:**
   a. There is a sound pathophysiological basis for prescribing a salt-free diet.
   b. Betahistine is a histamine agonist and vasodilator, which may improve stria vascularis ischaemia.
   c. Diuretic therapy improves the long-term course of the disease.
   d. Cinnarizine is a useful vestibular sedative.
   e. Streptomycin is useful as it has a purely vestibulotoxic effect.

106. *Synopsis 153–158; Scott-Brown 3/1/17, 3/19/18–24*
   a. False   Caloric responses are usually paretic; a directional preponderance to either side may be seen. Normal responses can occur during in the remission phase.
   b. False   The test depends upon the demonstration of an improvement in hearing thresholds. If they are nearly normal, it would be difficult to improve them further. It is most useful in those patients with fluctuating hearing loss. If in remission, the test is unreliable.
   c. True   Speech discrimination in cochlear deafness is usually better than in neural deafness with similar pure tone thresholds.
   d. True   This classically shows a large summating potential and an abnormal cochlear microphonic. The sensitivity of the test is enhanced by administration of acetazolamide (hydration). Electrical changes are reduced with glycerol (dehydration). In unilateral cases, the test may reveal the contralateral ear to be affected.
   e. False   This is a research investigation. If performed, the aqueduct is shown to be narrowed.

107. *Synopsis 157; Scott-Brown 2/6/15–17, 3/19/27 29*
   a. False   Nevertheless, some patients do appear to benefit from restriction of salt intake.
   b. True   However, this is not necessarily its mode of action in practice. The drug may also have effects on the vestibular nuclei.
   c. False   Diuretics are used to reproduce the improvement seen by the osmotic/diuretic effect of glycerol, but do not alter the long-term prognosis.
   d. True   It has both phenothiazine (antiemetic) and antihistamine properties.
   e. False   There is a danger of cochlear injury, particularly in the presence of inadequate renal function.

108. **Surgical management of Ménière's disease:**
    a. Vertiginous symptoms are least likely to be ameliorated.
    b. Georges Portmann was the first to perform a saccus endolymphaticus drainage procedure.
    c. An endolymphatic perilymphatic shunt can be created by cochleostomy.
    d. Vestibular nerve section can be performed via middle fossa, posterior fossa and supralabyrinthine approaches.
    e. A membranous labyrinthectomy carries the cost of losing the residual hearing in the operated ear.

109. **Pathology of presbyacusis:**
    a. Sensory presbyacusis is characterized by atrophy of the organ of Corti in the basal turn of the cochlea.
    b. A reduction in the number of cochlear spiral ganglion cells to 2000 produces a minimal effect on speech reception.
    c. A flat, pure tone audiometric curve is usually seen in cochlear conductive presbyacusis.
    d. The middle ear function plays a significant role in the audiometric changes.
    e. The rate of degeneration has an inherited predisposition.

108. *Synopsis 157–158; Scott-Brown 3/19/29–36*
  a. False   Most surgical procedures are designed to relieve
             vertigo. They may also prevent further hearing
             losses of a permanent nature.
  b. True   This was carried out in 1926. It would appear that
             the sac merely requires to be exposed, without
             incision and drainage, to produce benefit.
  c. True   Using an angled pick, inserted via the round
             window, the scala tympani (perilymph) and scala
             media (endolymph) are connected by puncturing
             the basilar membrane. This was devised by H. F.
             Schuknecht. The high risk of sensorineural hearing
             loss has discouraged its use.
  d. True.
  e. True   This can be performed either by fenestration of the
             lateral semicircular canal or by elevating the stapes
             footplate.

109. *Synopsis 158; Scott-Brown 2/10/19–20, 3/4/33–36*
  a. True   This explains the abrupt high tone loss. Speech
             discrimination remains satisfactory late in the
             process.
  b. False   There is a severe loss of speech discrimination, as
             found in neural presbyacusis. The ganglion cell
             population is normally 30 000.
  c. False   Strial atrophy produces a flat curve with a
             reasonable speech discrimination score. Cochlear
             conductive presbyacusis, probably due to changes
             in the motion mechanics of the basilar membrane,
             produces a descending audiometric pattern for
             bone conduction.
  d. False   Although thickening of the eardrum and ankylosis
             and laxity of ossicular articulation has been
             reported, there is only a minimal effect on hearing
             thresholds.
  e. True.

110. **Management of presbyacusis:**
    a. Sibilant and fricative consonants are well heard.
    b. The patient is more likely to understand the raised loud voice.
    c. Electronic hearing aids are the mainstay of treatment.
    d. Lip reading and auditory training are useful adjuncts.
    e. Amplification within the dynamic range provides better voice intelligibility.

111. **Ototoxic effects:**
    a. The effects of streptomycin are predominantly vestibulotoxic.
    b. The effects of neomycin may be delayed weeks or months following administration.
    c. The effects of salicylates are irreversible.
    d. The effects of anticonvulsant drugs can cause toxic effects on the vestibular system.
    e. The effects of diuretics are usually permanent.

110. *Synopsis 159; Scott-Brown 2/13/1–36, 2/14/1–27*
   a. False   They are poorly heard, as the high frequency tones are usually lost early in the process.
   b. False   Increased intensity may produce recruitment. The voice should be clearly articulated and normal in character, and spoken close to the patient's ear.
   c. True   Hearing aids with low tone cut and automatic volume control facilities are particularly useful.
   d. True   However, these are not easily mastered by the elderly.
   e. True   However, amplification to levels above the patient's loudness discomfort level results in distortion and reduced intelligibility.

111. *Synopsis 159–160; Scott-Brown 2/8/15–16, 3/20/1–15*
   a. True   However, with high doses and prolonged treatment, cochleotoxic effects are seen. The drug has been used in bilateral Ménière's disease to ablate vestibular function.
   b. True   The same applies with dihydrostreptomycin. All the aminoglycosides may exhibit this feature.
             Neomycin has a predominantly cochleotoxic effect.
   c. False   Tinnitus and/or hearing loss are usually reversible. Aetiology is a probably vasoconstriction of the cochlear microcirculation. Prostaglandins are implicated.
   d. True   Phenytoin in particular may produce a 'posterior fossa syndrome'. Cerebellar degeneration has been shown with chronic administration. Ethosuximide has similar vestibulotoxic side effects.
   e. False   Both ethacrynic acid and frusemide usually produce a temporary sensorineural deafness on intravenous administration. It may, rarely, be permanent.

112. **Tinnitus:**
   a. Palatal myoclonus may cause clicking noises, audible to the examining clinician.
   b. A glomus tumour is the commonest cause of pulsatile tinnitus.
   c. Pitch matching and loudness matching are essential techniques in the assessment of tinnitus.
   d. Ablative surgery of the auditory nerve is the treatment of choice for severe intractable tinnitus.
   e. Depression is the most commonly associated psychiatric condition.

113. **Cochlear implants:**
   a. A multichannel intracochlear electrode gives better speech discrimination results than a single channel extracochlear electrode.
   b. Deaf children should be implanted as young as possible because neuronal plasticity for speech development is significantly impaired by the age of 3 years.
   c. Post-lingually deafened candidates have better overall outcomes than those pre-lingually deafened.
   d. Pre-operative high resolution imaging is essential to detect bony obliteration of the cochlea or congenital abnormalities.
   e. Failure of treatment may be due to lack of spiral ganglion cell survival.

112. *Synopsis 165–166; Scott-Brown 2/18/1–34*
 a. True   This is a relative rarity.
 b. False   Glomus tumours are rare, pulsatile tinnitus is common and may or may not be associated with abnormalities of blood flow in vessels close to the ear.
 c. False   Only pure tone audiometry is essential. Pitch matching is of limited value, as many tinnitus sounds have no set pitch. Loudness matching (in terms of dB above threshold) is also of limited value, because many patients with tinnitus also suffer from recruitment.
 d. False   Indeed, this may make tinnitus worse.
 e. True.

113. *Synopsis 70–72; Scott-Brown 2/15/1–20, 3/25/1–20, 6/2/23, 6/11/1–15*
 a. True   Single channel devices were important in the early years of implantation, but are now virtually obsolete.
 b. True   It disappears entirely by the age of 6–8 years.
 c. True.
 d. True   CT, MRI or both can be used.
 e. True.

The nose and sinuses

1. **Blood supply of the nose:**
   a. Branches of both internal and external carotid arteries supply the nasal mucosa.
   b. The maxillary artery provides the major blood supply to the nasal fossa.
   c. Little's area is supplied by branches of the greater palatine, sphenopalatine, posterior ethmoidal and superior labial arteries.
   d. There is venous communication with the superior sagittal sinus via the foramen caecum.
   e. Sympathetic motor fibres controlling the mucosal vessels run in the Vidian nerve.

2. **Nasal anatomy:**
   a. The cell bodies of olfactory neurones lie in the nasal mucosa.
   b. The greater palatine nerve supplies most of the inferior turbinate with common sensation.
   c. The posterior lateral nasal nerves are branches of the posterior ethmoidal nerve.
   d. Lymph from the anterior part of the nose drains to the submental nodes.
   e. The posterior part of the nasal cavity drains to the retropharyngeal and upper deep cervical lymph nodes.

The nose and sinuses

1. *Synopsis 180–182; Scott-Brown 1/5/13–14, 4/18/1–5*
   a. True   The maxillary artery is an end branch of the external
            carotid; the internal carotid supplies blood to the
            superior part of the nose via the anterior and posterior
            ethmoidal branches of its ophthalmic branch.
   b. True   90 per cent of the nasal mucosa is supplied from the
            maxillary artery, and transantral ligation is an effective
            treatment for severe epistaxis.
   c. False This area is supplied by branches of the anterior
            ethmoidal artery.
   d. True   The foramen caecum lies in front of the crista galli,
            and transmits an emissary vein from the nose to the
            superior sagittal sinus.
   e. True   Both sympathetic and parasympathetic fibres run in
            the Vidian nerve, from the internal carotid plexus and
            greater superficial petrosal nerve respectively. The
            main effect of Vidian neurectomy, however, is to
            abolish parasympathetic overactivity.

2. *Synopsis 183–184; Scott-Brown 1/5/10–25*
   a. True   They are bipolar cells with non-medullated central
            processes terminating in the olfactory bulb.
   b. True   The lateral branch of the anterior ethmoidal nerve
            supplies the remainder.
   c. False They are branches of the sphenopalatine
            (pterygopalatine) ganglion.
   d. False It drains to the submandibular nodes.
   e. True   The fact that retropharyngeal nodes are often involved
            in spread of posterior nasal and nasopharyngeal
            tumours makes radical neck dissection a poor
            treatment, since the intervening retropharyngeal nodes
            cannot be excised.

3. **Examination of the nose and sinuses:**
   a. The superior turbinate is easily seen in a child by turning up the tip of the nose with the thumb.
   b. Application of vasoconstrictor solutions is contraindicated in the examination of the nose.
   c. Eustachian tube orifices can usually be seen clearly with a 4 mm diameter, 30° angle rigid endoscope passed along the floor of the nose.
   d. The middle meatus should normally be entered anteriorly by displacing the middle turbinate medially with the tip of the 4 mm diameter rigid nasendoscope.
   e. B-mode ultrasound scanning is the most accurate method of diagnosing maxillary sinusitis.

4. **Imaging of the paranasal sinuses:**
   a. In plain X-rays, the maxillary antrum is best seen in an occipitomental view (OMV).
   b. Coronal CT scans of the paranasal sinuses show the ostiomeatal complex in better detail than MRI.
   c. A concha bullosa cannot be identified on an axial CT scan.
   d. A fronto-ethmoidal mucocoele shows on CT as an expansile lesion extending into the orbit.
   e. Plain X-rays are of no value in the diagnosis of malignant neoplasms of the nose and sinuses.

The nose and sinuses

3. *Synopsis 184–188; Scott-Brown 4/1/1–8*
   a. False   Only the inferior and middle turbinates will be seen. This is the correct technique for examining the nose in a child.
   b. False   Vasoconstrictors are very useful in this situation, and are necessary for endoscopic examination.
   c. True   A flexible fibreoptic nasolaryngoscope is an alternative. Mirror examination of the nasopharynx has been largely superseded by endoscopic techniques.
   d. False   This manoeuvre would cause pain and possibly bleeding, and is not recommended routinely. The middle meatus is best entered posteriorly by rotating a 30° endoscope under the free posterior margin of the middle turbinate, then slowly withdrawing it while angulating it supero-laterally. A 2.7 mm diameter endoscope is preferable to a 4 mm one if the nose is narrow.
   e. False   Antroscopy is the most accurate method. Prior to sinus endoscopy, antral puncture and lavage was the 'gold standard', but false negatives were common. Plain X-rays carry a high false positive rate. Coronal CT scanning provides more precise information, but is expensive and gives too high a radiation dose to be recommended for routine diagnostic purposes.

4. *Synopsis 186–188; Scott-Brown 1/17/1–21, 4/3/1–22, 6/17/4*
   a. True   In an OMV the head is tilted backwards by about 20° to lift the maxillary antrum clear of the dense shadow of the petrous temporal bone.
   b. True   Demonstration of the ostiomeatal complex requires fine bone detail, an area where CT has the advantage.
   c. False   Pneumatization of the middle turbinate can be seen on both axial and coronal cuts, but the standard protocols for FESS involve much thinner slices so the abnormality is more likely to be identified on coronal sections.
   d. True   The globe may be displaced anteriorly, laterally and inferiorly. Other features of chronic rhinosinusitis, polyposis and previous surgery may additionally be present.
   e. False   Plain X-rays may occasionally show bone destruction and raise the suspicion of malignancy in cases where the history and clinical findings would otherwise be consistent with chronic inflammatory disease. CT and MRI are, of course, superior to plain films and are needed to plan treatment, but it is not appropriate to scan all patients with rhinological symptoms. Plain films retain a place as a first-line investigation.

5. **Surgical anatomy of the paranasal sinuses:**
    a.   The uncinate process is a crescentic projection of bone on the lateral nasal wall, lateral to the head of the middle turbinate.
    b.   The area below and lateral to the attachment of the middle turbinate is the 'danger area' in intranasal surgery.
    c.   The lateral wall of the ethmoidal labyrinth is relatively thick and is unlikely to be penetrated except by excessive force.
    d.   If meningitis follows intranasal surgery, the cribriform plate must have been penetrated.
    e.   Onodi cells are posterior ethmoid cells lateral to the sphenoid, and may increase the risk of optic nerve damage.

6. **Antral puncture and lavage:**
    a.   This is usually performed through the middle meatus.
    b.   In children under 3 years of age, it is best performed through the canine fossa.
    c.   A second cannula may be required if the ostium is blocked.
    d.   It may be carried out as a diagnostic or a therapeutic manoeuvre.
    e.   The opening into the sinus is permanent.

7. **Paranasal sinus operations:**
    a.   The Caldwell-Luc operation (sublabial antrostomy) includes routine division of the descending palatine artery.
    b.   Inferior meatal antrostomy relies upon gravitational drainage and aeration to effect improvement in the sinus mucosa, while mucociliary clearance continues toward the natural ostium.
    c.   Lynch-Howarth external fronto-ethmoidectomy can be complicated by late formation of a mucocoele.
    d.   The sphenoidal sinus can be approached by intranasal and transantral routes, external ethmoidectomy, transpalatal and trans-septal routes.
    e.   The ethmoidal sinuses can be widely exposed in lateral rhinotomy.

5. *Synopsis 188–192; Scott-Brown 4/12/3–5*
   a. True   It is the site for the first incision in a Messerklinger infundibulotomy.
   b. False The 'danger areas' are above, lateral and medial to the vertical attachment of the middle turbinate.
   c. False The lamina papyracea forms the lateral border of the ethmoid and the medial orbital wall. As the name implies, it is paper-thin.
   d. False Infection can spread via the perineural lymphatics of the olfactory nerve filaments, and via the roof of the ethmoids.
   e. True   The optic nerve is at risk in any ethmoid surgery, but anatomical variants may increase the risk.

6. *Synopsis 189; Scott Brown 4/12/7–9*
   a. False The inferior meatus is more commonly used. The middle meatus carries a risk of subsequent stenosis of the ostium, and the orbit is more easily entered.
   b. False This is hazardous due to the presence of unerupted teeth in the wall. It is very rarely required in children.
   c. True.
   d. True   However, its diagnostic role is now greatly diminished because of the advent of nasal sinus endoscopy.
   e. False Even the large defect created by a formal antrostomy tends to close over.

7. *Synopsis 188 192; Scott-Brown 4/12/7–29*
   a. False The opening of the nasal antrostomy into the inferior meatus should not extend too far posteriorly, or the descending branches of the sphenopalatine and greater palatine arteries will be damaged, with severe haemorrhage.
   b. True   The inferior meatal antrostomy is being superseded by endoscopic middle meatal surgery, largely on the basis that this appears to be a more 'physiological' approach.
   c. True   The operation comprises removal of the floor of the frontal sinus and the anterior ethmoidal cells to create a wide passage into the middle meatus. However, stenosis may occur, leading to mucocoele formation.
   d. True.
   e. True.

8. **Nasal respiration:**
   a. Neonates are obligate nose breathers.
   b. Nasal breathing stops reflexively during swallowing.
   c. The anterior end of the inferior turbinate is important in regulating inspiratory airflow.
   d. Expiratory air currents are determined solely by the state of the posterior choanae.
   e. Eddy currents under the middle turbinate help provide conditioned air around the sinus ostia.

9. **The mucociliary 'conveyor belt' of the upper respiratory tract:**
   a. The cilia beat 100 times a second.
   b. The movement directs the mucus to the anterior nares.
   c. Lysozymes are produced by bacteria and act to paralyse cilia.
   d. A deviated nasal septum can produce localized drying with ciliary stasis, crusting and secondary infection.
   e. Ephedrine 0.5 per cent nose drops cause ciliary damage.

10. **Anosmia:**
   a It must be bilateral before it is noticeable.
   b. It is often described as loss of taste.
   c. It can be tested for by simple objective methods.
   d. It may be due to a brain tumour.
   e. Recovery usually occurs after skull fracture, beginning about 12 months after the injury.

8. *Synopsis 193–194; Scott-Brown 1/6/1–5, 4/4/1–15*
   a. True Congenital bilateral choanal atresia presents as a
   neonate who fails to breathe until distressed, and is
   then able to breathe through the mouth while crying.
   When crying ceases, the cycle repeats itself.
   Emergency treatment is provision of an oral airway.
   b. True.
   c. True It acts by varying the degree of engorgement of the
   venous plexuses in the submucosal erectile tissue.
   d. False These are determined by the dynamic anatomy of the
   entire nasal passage.
   e. True.

9 *Synopsis 195–197; Scott-Brown 1/6/5–10*
   a. False They beat 10 times a second.
   b. False The mucus is directed to the nasopharynx.
   c. False Lysozymes are protective bacteriolytic enzymes
   produced by the nasal mucosa.
   d. True Drying may be localized, or generalized due to
   constant exposure to dry air (e.g. central heating).
   e. False However, prolonged use of any vasoconstrictor will
   cause rebound congestion and may result in chronic
   hypertrophic rhinitis (rhinitis medicamentosa).

10. *Synopsis 197; Scott-Brown 1/6/16–19, 4/5/3–7*
   a. True.
   b. True Flavours are mainly perceived by olfaction.
   c. False Simple methods such as test solutions of, for example,
   lemon or cloves require subjective responses and are
   unreliable. Objective testing methods such as electro-
   olfactography and positron emission tomography are
   complex, difficult and imperfectly developed.
   d. True This is particularly so with frontal lobe lesions.
   e. False Where anosmia follows skull fracture, recovery is
   unlikely if it has not begun within 3 months.

11. **Disorders of smell:**
    a. Hyposmia can be caused by rhinitis in the absence of mechanical obstruction.
    ✓ b. Where influenza causes a peripheral olfactory neuritis, the loss of smell is usually permanent.
    c. Cacosmia may be due to a foreign body in the nose.
    d. Temporal lobe epilepsy may cause olfactory hallucinations.
    e. Ammonia is used to stimulate the olfactory nerve in suspected malingerers.

12. **Cleft lip and cleft palate:**
    a. The cleft lip results from failure of fusion of the maxillary process with the median nasal process.
    b. Flattening of the nostril is a feature.
    c. The nasal septum may be abnormally thick.
    d. The deformities result from teratogenic or genetic factors operating in the second month of foetal life.
    e. Bifid uvula is a minor form.

13. **Congenital nasal malformations:**
    a. A midline dermoid cyst should be distinguished from a meningocoele at operation.
    b. Dermoid cysts may present as a hairy fistula.
    c. Aplasia of the maxillary sinus is as common as aplasia of the frontal sinus.
    d. Exorbitism is a feature of Crouzon's syndrome.
    e. Atresia of the anterior nares is common in those of black African origin.

✓ 14. **Congenital choanal atresia:**
    a. This is most commonly a membranous closure.
    b. It is most commonly bilateral.
    c. It occurs more often in females.
    d. If unilateral, it tends to present late with persistent watery rhinorrhoea.
    e. Bilateral cases may be fatal.

11. *Synopsis 197–199; Scott-Brown 4/5/1–8*
    a. True   It is caused particularly by long-standing intrinsic or vasomotor rhinitis.
    b. True.
    c. True   Cacosmia is the perception of a bad smell due to an intrinsic cause.
    d. True.
    e. False Ammonia stimulates the trigeminal nerve. It is used to test for psychogenic causes.

12. *Synopsis 200–201; Scott-Brown 2/19/10–35*
    a. True.
    b. True   This is especially so in cases of bilateral cleft lip.
    c. True.
    d. True.
    e. True.

13. *Synopsis 200–204; Scott-Brown 6/15/1–10, 6/16/1–52*
    a. False The distinction should be made pre-operatively.
    b. True   The fistula may extend intracranially.
    c. False Failure of pneumatization is not uncommon in the frontal sinus, but is rare in the maxillary sinus.
    d. True   Crouzon's syndrome is a form of craniofacial dysostosis, characterized by calvarial deformity, mid-face hypoplasia and exorbitism.
    e.   False It is rare in all races.

14. *Synopsis 202–204; Scott-Brown 6/15/2–5*
    a. False Most are bony.
    b. False Unilateral congenital choanal atresia is commoner, occurring in 60 per cent of cases.
    c. True   The ratio of female to male is 2:1.
    d. False Late presentation is the rule, but the nasal discharge is thick and tenacious.
    e. True   The neonate is an obligate nasal breather. Failure to provide an oral airway can result in death from asphyxia. It may be associated with other serious congenital abnormalities such as cardiac anomalies.

15. **Management of maxillofacial injuries:**
    a. The first consideration is to look for signs of shock.
    b. The patient should be positioned supine.
    c. X-rays are the most useful diagnostic manoeuvre.
    d. Nasal obstruction indicates septal dislocation or haematoma.
    e. Serial neurological observations should be recorded.

16. **Middle-third facial fractures:**
    a. A Le Fort I (Guérin) fracture involves the orbit.
    b. Malocclusion is common.
    c. Trismus is due to associated temporomandibular joint dislocation.
    d. Epiphora indicates involvement of the nasolacrimal duct.
    e. An opaque antrum on X-ray is an indication for antral puncture and lavage.

17. **Blowout fracture of the orbit:**
    a. This may be caused by using excessive force when blowing the nose.
    b. The eyeball herniates into the antrum.
    c. The patient is unable to look down.
    d. Treatment should be delayed until oedema has settled if the forced duction test shows marked limitation of movement.
    e. Silastic sheeting is a suitable material for repair of the orbital floor.

18. **Fractures involving the frontal or ethmoidal sinuses:**
    a. CSF rhinorrhoea implies a dural tear.
    b. Nose blowing may cause an intracranial aerocoele.
    c. Systemic antibiotics are routinely given to prevent meningitis.
    d. If the posterior wall of the frontal sinus alone is involved and there is no aerocoele, early repair is unnecessary.
    e. A fascial graft may be used to repair a dural tear.

15. *Synopsis 204–207; Scott-Brown 4/16/1–10*
    a. False   The first consideration is the airway.
    b. False   The patient should be in the recovery position.
    c. False   The diagnosis can usually be made clinically. X-rays are mainly of medicolegal importance.
    d. True   Septal haematoma requires urgent drainage.
    e. True   Observations should be recorded using a standard chart such as the Glasgow coma scale.

16. *Synopsis 207–209; Scott-Brown 1/8/8, 4/16/4–22*
    a. False   The Le Fort I fracture passes below the orbit. Types II and III do involve the orbit.
    b. True   This is one of the main diagnostic features. It requires skilled treatment by an oral surgeon.
    c. False   Trismus is due to a combination of malocclusion and soft tissue swelling.
    d. True.
    e. False   An opaque antrum is caused by blood, and does not require lavage.

17. *Synopsis 210; Scott-Brown 4/16/3, 25, 4/24/10–11*
    a. False   The cause is a backward blow on the eyeball.
    b. False   Orbital fat, with or without the inferior rectus muscle, herniates into the antrum.
    c. False   Upward gaze is limited, resulting in vertical diplopia. Other eye movements are usually unaffected.
    d. False   Treatment should be carried out as soon as possible if diplopia is to be avoided.
    e. True.

18. *Synopsis 210–211; Scott-Brown 4/16/9–27*
    a. True   This may be difficult to detect early because of bleeding.
    b. True   This is commonest if the lamina papyracea is fractured.
    c. True   Penicillin and sulphadimidine are the traditional choice.
    d. True   The indication for early fascial repair is intracranial aerocoele. A persistent CSF leak may require late repair.
    e. True   Other materials are also used, such as collagen felt and tissue glue.

19. **Cerebrospinal fluid rhinorrhoea:**
    a. The usual symptom is clear, watery fluid dripping from the nose.
    b. The fluid contains glucose.
    c. The site of the leak is determined by clinical examination.
    d. Initial treatment is to pack the nose with BIPP.
    e. Endonasal endoscopic repair carries less morbidity than craniotomy, and is the treatment of choice where the leak is clearly localized and has failed to respond to conservative measures.

20. **Oro-antral fistula:**
    a. Dental extraction is the usual cause of the alveolar type of oro-antral fistula.
    b. Regurgitation of food into the nose is a symptom.
    c. Maxillary sinusitis frequently ensues.
    d. Intranasal antrostomy is part of the treatment.
    e. The rim of a sublabial fistula should be excised.

21. **Bullet wounds to the head and neck region:**
    a. High-velocity missile wounds are less likely to be contaminated than those caused by low-velocity missiles.
    b. Damage far from the path of the bullet may be caused by a travelling shock wave.
    c. The first principle of treatment is to excise devitalized tissue.
    d. Primary closure is contraindicated.
    e. Fixation of facial fractures is unnecessary.

19. *Synopsis 211; Scott-Brown 4/12/25, 4/14/1–12, 4/16/26–27*
a. True   Some cases present with meningitis.
b. True   Fluid is tested using dextrostix.
c. False   Clinical examination can rarely determine the site of
           the leak. High-resolution coronal CT scanning is the
           most useful method, together with rigid nasal
           endoscopy. Intrathecal fluorescein and the use of a
           blue light increase the sensitivity of endoscopic
           examination.
d. False   This would be extremely dangerous and could lead to
           meningitis. Treatment initially consists of prophylactic
           antibiotics, with strict avoidance of nose-blowing or
           any local interference.
e. True.

20. *Synopsis 212; Scott-Brown 4/22/9*
a. True   Other causes are erosion by malignancy, and
           penetrating wounds. Caldwell-Luc and similar
           operations may cause a sublabial fistula.
b. True   Regurgitation of air and fluid is more common.
c. True   The infection tends to produce particularly foul-
           smelling pus with dental cases.
d. True   This allows drainage into the nose. A general principle
           of treatment for any fistula is to provide proximal
           drainage.
e. True   The mucosal edges are then undercut and sutured.

21. *Synopsis 213; Scott-Brown 4/16/1 6*
a. False   A high-velocity missile causes a large cavity to form
           and the vacuum sucks in dirt and organisms from the
           skin.
b. True   The intima of the carotid artery may be lifted up in this
           way.
c. False   Devitalized tissue should be excised, but the first
           principle of treatment is to safeguard the airway.
d. False   Primary closure can be undertaken in this region
           because of the excellent blood supply.
e. False   Fixation may be essential.

22. **Sinus barotrauma:**
    a. This is due to excessively high pressure in the sinus.
    b. It is more likely to occur in the presence of an upper respiratory tract infection.
    c. Pain is usually felt during descent.
    d. Submucosal haemorrhage is a pathological feature.
    e. Decongestant nasal drops are helpful prophylactically.

23. **Nasal septal deformities:**
    a. These may be caused by birth trauma.
    b. A deviated septum is associated with high arched palate.
    c. A spur predisposes to epistaxes.
    d. Submucous resection (SMR) is the treatment of choice in children.
    e. Septoplasty aims to conserve but straighten septal cartilage and bone.

24. **Septal haematomas:**
    a. Septal haematomas are usually traumatic in origin.
    b. They may be due to a blood dyscrasia.
    c. Unilateral nasal obstruction is the commonest symptom.
    d. They are likely to resolve spontaneously without complication.
    e. Treatment is conservative unless an abscess develops.

22. *Synopsis 213; Scott-Brown 1/7/17–19*
  a. False It is due to low pressure in the sinus.
  b. True This is because the sinus ostium is more likely to be obstructed, preventing pressure equalization.
  c. True.
  d. True Earlier changes are mucosal congestion, inflammation, oedema, and haemorrhage. Submucosal haemorrhage occurs in severe cases.
  e. True However, they are not suitable for long-term use.

23. *Synopsis 214–215; Scott-Brown 1/5/2–4, 4/11/1–27*
  a. True However, this is a rare cause. Most are due to trauma later in life.
  b. True The congenital high-arched palate leaves less room for the vertical height of the septum, which tends to buckle.
  c. True Bleeding occurs from vessels crossing its sharp convex surface.
  d. False Children are treated either by expectant management, waiting until they are around 16 years of age, or by conservative septoplasty. Standard SMR is likely to produce deformity of growth.
  e. True.

24. *Synopsis 215; Scott-Brown 4/11/1–2, 4/16/3–4*
  a. True Trauma may be external or surgical.
  b. True.
  c. False Bilateral obstruction is the most common symptom.
  d. False Septal abscess and subsequent cartilage necrosis are likely to occur. In the absence of infection, permanent gross thickening of the septum is likely.
  e. False The haematoma should be evacuated, provision for drainage made, and nasal splints and/or packs inserted to prevent a further accumulation. Systemic antibiotics are prescribed to prevent secondary infection.

25. **Septal abscess:**
    a. A septal abscess is always secondary to a septal haematoma.
    b. Pain is localized to the tip of the nose.
    c. Systemic symptoms are unusual.
    d. A septal perforation may ensue.
    e. Initial treatment consists of incision and drainage plus systemic antibiotics.

26. **Septal perforation:**
    a. Most cases are due to nose-picking, syphilis or cocaine abuse.
    b. Chromic acid is a recognized industrial cause.
    c. Large perforations characteristically cause a whistling noise.
    d. The cartilaginous septum is most commonly involved, except in syphilitic cases, when it is the bony septum.
    e. Surgical repair is usually advisable because of the danger of severe epistaxes.

27. **Foreign bodies in the nose:**
    a. These usually present in adult life.
    b. Epistaxis is the commonest clinical feature.
    c. Non-organic materials cause more tissue reaction than organic.
    d. A bead should be removed with non-toothed dissecting forceps.
    e. General anaesthetic is often required in children.

25. *Synopsis 215–216; Scott-Brown 4/11/2*
 a. False A septal abscess may also follow a nasal furuncle or occur spontaneously in the course of childhood exanthemata.
 b. False Severe generalized headache is the commonest type of pain associated with a septal abscess. The nose is locally tender.
 c. False The patient is generally unwell, with fever.
 d. True Cartilage necrosis may also occur with subsequent nasal collapse. Rarely, cavernous sinus thrombosis or meningitis ensues.
 e. True.

26. *Synopsis 216; Scott-Brown 4/11/18–25*
 a. False The majority of cases are traumatic in origin, usually following septal surgery.
 b. True Chrome is used in metal plating; also in tanning, dyeing and some photographic processes.
 c. False Small perforations cause whistling.
 d. True.
 e. False Many cases are asymptomatic and require no treatment. Conservative treatment is usual; for example, glucose and glycerin drops to prevent crusting. Epistaxis from septal perforation is usually minor, and follows separation of crusts. A silastic 'button' can be used or surgical repair carried out, but results are unreliable.

27. *Synopsis 217–219; Scott-Brown 6/14/3–6*
 a. False These are much commoner in children.
 b. False Patients either present acutely with a known foreign body, or with a chronic unilateral nasal discharge.
 c. False Organic materials cause severe mucosal inflammation.
 d. False A bead should be removed with a blunt hook. Forceps are likely to push the foreign body deeper into the nose.
 e. True No attempt should be made to remove a foreign body in an uncooperative child.

28. Rhinolith:
   a. A rhinolith is a stony, hard nose, caused by infiltration with tumour.
   b. Rhinoliths can be formed from organized blood clots.
   c. They are characterized by extreme pain.
   d. They can often be detected using a probe.
   e. Rhinoliths are radio-opaque.

29. Inflammation of the external nose:
   a. Furunculosis arises from a staphylococcal infection of a pilosebaceous follicle in the vestibule.
   b. Cavernous sinus thrombosis may complicate furunculosis.
   c. Painful fissures occur in chronic vestibulitis.
   d. Erysipelas is an acute, spreading staphylococcal dermatitis.
   e. Acne rosacea may progress to rhinophyma.

30. Acute infective rhinitis:
   a. This is most commonly caused by the rhinovirus.
   b. A green discharge indicates secondary bacterial infection.
   c. Otitis media is a common complication in children.
   d. Vasoconstrictor nose drops should not be used.
   e. Vaccination provides effective protection.

28. *Synopsis 218–219; Scott-Brown 6/14/4–6*
    a. False A rhinolith is a concretion of calcium and magnesium salts which builds up, over many years, around a foreign body in the nasal fossa. It can also form around inspissated mucus or blood clot (endogenous rhinolith).
    b. True.
    c. False Unilateral nasal obstruction and discharge are the characteristic symptoms. Some rhinoliths go unrecognized for many years.
    d. True A grating sensation is felt.
    e. True This is because of the calcification.

29. *Synopsis 219–221; Scott-Brown 4/2/1–9, 4/8/21*
    a. True However, between 25 and 40 per cent of normal individuals may carry *Staphylococcus aureus* in the vestibule without symptoms.
    b. True This rarely occurs in the antibiotic era. Squeezing the pustules may encourage venous embolism of bacteria to the cavernous sinus.
    c. True The fissures are treated by barrier cream with topical antibiotic or antiseptic.
    d. False It is streptococcal. *Staphylococcus* causes impetigo rather than erysipelas.
    e. True.

30. *Synopsis 221–223; Scott-Brown 4/8/13–19*
    a. True.
    b. True Organisms include *Streptococcus pneumoniae*, *Staphylococcus aureus*, *Haemophilus influenzae*, and *Klebsiella* spp.
    c. True The middle ear mucosa is an extension of the upper respiratory tract.
    d. False They provide effective symptomatic relief of nasal obstruction, and may prevent the complication of sinusitis. However, they should not be used for longer than a week.
    e. False There are so many different viruses that cause the condition (at least 200), it is not feasible to vaccinate against all of them. Influenza vaccines are used to protect patients at special risk, e.g. chronic bronchitics, but vaccines only protect against specific strains of influenza virus.

31. **Chronic non-specific rhinitis:**
    a. Aetiological factors include atmospheric pollution and excessive dryness.
    b. A deviated nasal septum is a predisposing factor.
    c. The goblet cells increase, while ciliated cells are lost from the epithelium.
    d. Nasal obstruction commonly alternates from side to side.
    e. Inferior turbinectomy is the treatment of choice.

32. **Chronic hypertrophic rhinitis:**
    a. This can be caused by abuse of vasoconstrictor drops (rhinitis medicamentosa).
    b. The mucosa of the inferior turbinates is particularly affected.
    c. A mulberry turbinate may be seen prolapsing through the nostril.
    d. Fibrosis causing lymphatic obstruction may be a contributory factor in polyp formation.
    e. Treatment consists of oral antihistamines and local injection of sclerosants.

✓ 33. **Atrophic rhinitis:**
    a. The patient suffers from cacosmia.
    b. The primary form is commonest in young women.
    c. Syphilis should be excluded.
    d. Local treatment is with glucose 25 per cent in glycerin drops.
    e. Surgery to narrow the nasal airways may be effective.

31. *Synopsis 223–225; Scott-Brown 4/8/12, 4/8/23–25*
  a. True   The condition is multifactorial in origin.
  b. True   This is because a deviated nasal septum may cause localized areas of dryness and crusting, or interfere with normal drainage.
  c. True   The same as in chronic bronchitis.
  d. True   This is an exaggeration of the normal nasal cycle. When lying down, the dependent nostril is blocked.
  e. False Surgical treatment is reserved for cases where pathological changes are irreversible and/or medical treatment has failed.

32. *Synopsis 225; Scott-Brown 4/9/1–14, 4/10/2–3*
  a. True   It may also be simply an advanced case of chronic non-specific rhinitis.
  b. True   However, all areas of mucosa may show some changes.
  c. False The mulberry turbinate is the hypertrophied posterior end of the inferior turbinate, and is seen occupying the choana on mirror examination or endoscopy of the nasopharynx.
  d. True   This is a plausible theory, although the aetiology of nasal polyps is not fully understood.
  e. False Treatment consists of stopping any predisposing factors (e.g. vasoconstrictor abuse, smoking, alcohol abuse), attention to sinus infection and local treatment with a steroid spray, followed by surgical removal of chronically hypertrophied mucosa, straightening of septal deviations and polypectomy.

33. *Synopsis 226–227; Scott-Brown 4/8/26–27*
  a. False The patient has ozaena. Cacosmia is the perception of a bad smell in the nose due to an intrinsic cause. Although patients with atrophic rhinitis have a foul smell in the nose, they are themselves anosmic.
  b. True   Onset is often around the time of puberty.
  c. True.
  d. True   This follows removal of any crusts with warm isotonic saline or an alkaline nasal douche.
  e. True   Submucosal grafts, Teflon™ injections and suturing of the nostrils have all been advocated.

34. **Wegener's granulomatosis:**
    a. This affects the nose, lungs and kidney.
    b. It is fatal without treatment.
    c. The pathological lesion is similar to polyarteritis nodosa.
    d. The anti-neutrophil cytoplasmic antibody (ANCA) test is positive, and the ESR mirrors the clinical course of the disease.
    e. Combination steroid and cytotoxic therapy improves the survival rate compared to steroid treatment alone.

35. **Syphilis and the nose:**
    a. 'Snuffles' affects infants aged 2–5 years with congenital syphilis.
    b. Nasal chancre is associated with painful submaxillary lymphadenopathy.
    c. Secondary syphilis may masquerade as a persistent coryza.
    d. A gumma is the commonest nasal manifestation of syphilis.
    e. Serological tests are unlikely to be positive in tertiary syphilis.

36. **Nasal lupus vulgaris:**
    a. This is a tuberculous infection of the skin.
    b. The source is frequently pulmonary tuberculosis in a family member.
    c. 'Apple jelly' nodules are seen histologically.
    d. The cartilaginous septum may perforate.
    e. Antituberculous drugs promote rapid healing without deformity.

34. *Synopsis 227–228; Scott-Brown 4/2/7–8, 4/20/5–8*
  a. True   Other regions may also be involved, e.g. the ear or
          pharynx.
  b. True   Fatality may sometimes occur in a very short space of
          time – 24 hours in fulminant cases. Death is usually
          due to renal failure.
  c. True   Giant cells are also seen in the granulomata. However,
          histological confirmation of the disease may be
          difficult; frequently a clinical decision has to be made
          to start treatment.
  d. True   High levels of ANCA and a high ESR both reduce
          when the disease is treated or regresses.
  e. True   Azathioprine and cyclophosphamide are used, and
          have revolutionized the prognosis.

35. *Synopsis 228–229; Scott-Brown 4/2/3–4, 4/8/28–31, 4/20/2, 6/17/2*
  a. False   'Snuffles' affects the neonate, up to around 3 months.
          It can cause major difficulties with feeding.
  b. False   The lymphadenopathy is painless.
  c. True   Other manifestations should be looked for, e.g. snail-
          track ulcers, rash, generalized lymphadenopathy.
  d. True   It usually occurs in the bony septum, but any part of
          the nose may be affected.
  e. False   Approximately 90 per cent of tests will be positive.
          Serology is usually negative in primary syphilis.

36. *Synopsis 230; Scott-Brown 4/2/3, 4/8/30–32*
  a. True.
  b. True.
  c. False   'Apple jelly' nodules are seen clinically, by pressing on
          the affected skin with a glass slide. The histological
          appearances are typical of tuberculosis elsewhere,
          namely caseating granulomata with giant cell
          formation.
  d. True.
  e. False   Antituberculous drugs will arrest the course of the
          disease, but healing is by fibrosis and deformities will
          occur. Of course, any destruction of tissue that has
          already taken place cannot be reversed by drug
          treatment. Plastic reconstructive procedures will often
          be required.

37. Chronic specific rhinitis:
 a. Sarcoidosis usually presents as an atrophic ulcer.
 b. Yaws is the commonest cause of a runny nose in Jamaica.
 c. Leprosy causes excruciatingly painful ulceration.
 d. Rhinosporidiosis presents as a bleeding raspberry-like polyp.
 e. Nasopharyngeal Leishmaniasis is transmitted by the South American sandfly.

38. Acute infective sinusitis:
 a. This is usually caused by a preceding coryza.
 b. It can follow barotrauma.
 c. If secondary to dental infection, the causative organism is likely to be *Haemophilus influenzae*.
 d. There is initially reduced mucosal glandular secretion.
 e. An empyema is a collection of seromucinous fluid in the sinus.

39. Acute infective sinusitis:
 a. Pain is limited to the area overlying the affected sinus.
 b. Oedema of the overlying tissues is commoner in children.
 c. Mucopurulent nasal discharge is necessary to make the diagnosis.
 d. Decongestant nose drops are used to provide 'medical drainage'.
 e. An antibiotic solution should be instilled into the sinus cavity during antral lavage.

37. *Synopsis 228–233; Scott-Brown 4/8/26–39*
- a. False Nasal sarcoid usually presents as nodules or crusting on the septum, vestibule or anterior ends of inferior turbinates. It may also present as a lupus pernio. Widespread distribution is characteristic.
- b. False Although yaws is common in Jamaica, it rarely affects the nose.
- c. False Lepromatous ulceration is painless because the peripheral nerves are destroyed.
- d. True This is due to infection by the sporozoon *Rhinosporidium kinealyi* or *R. seeberi.*
- e. True The non-flagellated form of *Leishmania braziliensis* can be found in the discharge and in the granulomata.

38. *Synopsis 223–228; Scott-Brown 4/8/1–25*
- a. True.
- b. True.
- c. False Anaerobic organisms are characteristic of dental infection. *H. influenzae* causes epidemics of sinusitis, particularly in children.
- d. False There is hypersecretion.
- e. False The sinus contains infected mucopus.

39. *Synopsis 223–228; Scott-Brown 4/8/1–25*
- a. False Pain from sinusitis can radiate widely. Tenderness is usually localized over the affected sinus.
- b. True Swelling of the cheek occurs in maxillary sinusitis, and of the orbit in ethmoidal sinusitis.
- c. False The discharge is only present if the sinus is draining ('open' sinusitis). A 'closed' sinusitis can cause severe symptoms, but there is no mucopurulent discharge because the ostium is blocked.
- d. True Vasoconstriction of the congested nasal mucosa around the sinus ostia promotes drainage.
- e. False Systemic antibiotics are given. Washouts are usually performed with physiological saline.

40. Chronic non-specific sinusitis:

√   a.   This may be due to an unresolved attack of acute sinusitis.
      b.   Perennial non-allergic rhinitis is an aetiological factor in two out of three cases.
      c.   Multiple small abscesses in the thickened mucosa are recognized pathological features.
      d.   Bacteriology usually reveals pure cultures of streptococci.
      e.   A postnasal drip is a *sine qua non* for the diagnosis.

41. Chronic rhinosinusitis:

      a.   Eosinophils and polymorphonucleocytes may be found in the discharge.
      b.   The frontal sinus is most commonly affected.
      c.   Polyps are often found, and may block the sinus ostia.
      d.   Topical steroid therapy should be avoided because of the danger of uncontrolled infection.
      e.   A radical operation offers a good prospect of a permanent cure.

42. Acute maxillary sinusitis:

      a.   The infection is of dental origin in 1 per cent of cases.
      b.   Tenderness is usually localized over the sinus.
      c.   X-rays are of no value in the acute phase.
      d.   Antral washouts should be performed as soon as possible, to establish the diagnosis and commence treatment.
      e.   Toothache precedes sinusitis in all cases of an apical abscess.

40. *Synopsis 238–241; Scott-Brown 4/8/1–25*
a. True.
b. True.
c. True   The pathological appearances are variable, even within the individual patient. Polyps, atrophic mucosa, fibrosis, epithelial metaplasia, abscesses, cysts and granulations all occur.
d. False   Mixed growth is usual. Anaerobes are common. *Streptococcus pneumoniae* and Gram-negative bacilli often coexist.
e. False   Although postnasal drip is a very common symptom – and one of the most difficult to relieve – it is not necessary to make the diagnosis.

41. *Synopsis 241–242; Scott-Brown 4/8/1–25*
a. True   Eosinophils are especially prominent when there is an allergic component, polymorphonucleocytes when infection predominates.
b. False   The maxillary and ethmoidal sinuses are most commonly affected.
c. True.
d. False   Topical steroid therapy is one of the most effective forms of treatment, and has very few side effects. Antibiotics are indicated in the presence of active infection.
e. False   The condition is chronic and is unlikely to be completely cured by surgery. Septal and functional endoscopic sinus surgery has a role in providing an adequate airway, and in removing obstruction from the ostiomeatal complex to encourage restoration of mucociliary clearance.

42. *Synopsis 234–236; Scott-Brown 4/8/18–20*
a. False   Dental infection causes around 10 per cent of cases.
b. True   Although the pain can radiate widely, tenderness is usually localized.
c. False   X-rays are the main diagnostic investigation.
d. False   Antibiotics and nasal decongestants should be given first. If the response is unsatisfactory, antral washouts should be performed.
e. False   A dead tooth with an apical abscess can be painless.

⌡ **43. Acute frontal sinusitis:**
   a. The frontal sinus alone is usually affected.
   b. Pain is typically worse in the morning.
   c. Discharge is seen in the inferior meatus, where the fronto-nasal duct opens.
   d. Treatment is to cannulate the sinus via its natural ostium.
   e. Trephining the orbital roof should be avoided because of the danger of spreading infection to the eye.

44. Acute sphenoidal sinusitis:
   a. Acute sphenoidal sinusitis is not uncommon.
   b. The posterior ethmoidal cells are involved in most cases.
   c. Pain may simulate acute mastoiditis.
   d. Discharge is seen at the back of the nose.
   e. The sinus can be punctured and washed out transnasally.

45. Treatment of chronic maxillary sinusitis:
   a. Medical treatment is useless; surgery is nearly always required.
   b. Antral washouts should be performed daily for 3 weeks in the first instance.
   c. Messerklinger infundibulotomy commences by incising the anterior attachment of the uncinate process with a sickle knife.
   d. Middle meatal antrostomy can be performed with a Stammberger back-biting punch.
   e. The Caldwell-Luc operation involves enlarging the natural ostium to allow free drainage.

43. *Synopsis 236–237; Scott-Brown 4/8/18, 4/12/14*
   a. False   The anterior ethmoidal and maxillary sinuses are
             usually affected as well.
   b. True   It is often associated with swelling of the upper eyelid.
   c. False   The frontal recess opens into the middle meatus.
   d. False   Cannulation of the ostium via the frontal recess is
             difficult, and may cause damage with subsequent
             stenosis. Treatment consists of systemic antibiotics,
             local decongestants and treatment of concurrent
             ethmoidal and maxillary sinusitis. In cases that fail
             to settle promptly, the floor of the frontal sinus can
             be trephined via the orbital roof. Some advocate
             placing a plastic tube for irrigation until the infection
             is under control.
   e. False   See above.

44. *Synopsis 237; Scott-Brown 4/8/18*
   a. False   It is rare.
   b. True   Involvement is most commonly as part of a
             pansinusitis.
   c. True   Pain may radiate anywhere in the head.
   d. True.
   e. True   However, this is rarely performed.

45. *Synopsis 239; Scott-Brown 4/8/23–25, 4/12/10–24*
   a. False   Medical treatment is the mainstay of all forms of
             chronic sinusitis, particularly topical steroids. Surgery
             is now required much less frequently than in the past.
   b. False   Very few patients would tolerate this medieval regime.
   c. True   This is the first step in most FESS operations.
   d. True   Alternatively, an Ostrom punch may be used.
   e. False   The antrostomy is made into the inferior meatus.

46. **Treatment of chronic frontal sinusitis:**
    a. FESS with endoscopic dissection of the frontal recess is contraindicated because of the risk of spreading infection into the ethmoid.
    b. The Lynch-Howarth operation combines treatment of frontal and maxillary sinuses.
    c. A drainage tube is left in the nose for several weeks after the Howarth operation.
    d. Obliteration of the sinus is an alternative to a drainage procedure.
    e. An osteoplastic flap is hinged superiorly.

47. **Aetiology of sinusitis in children:**
    a. Antibody deficiency is a common cause of sinusitis in children.
    b. Dietary deficiency and poor social conditions are contributory.
    c. Bacteriology usually shows a pure growth of *Haemophilus influenzae* in chronic cases.
    d. Childhood exanthemata may initiate chronic sinusitis.
    ✓ e. Kartagener's syndrome consists of sinusitis, bronchitis and congenital cyanotic heart disease.

48. **Sinusitis in children:**
    a. The frontal sinus is poorly developed before the fifth year of life.
    b. In acute sinusitis, oedema of the cheeks and eyelids is commoner in children than adults.
    c. Pain is the principal clinical feature of chronic sinusitis in children.
    d. Chronic ethmoidal sinusitis should be treated as soon as it is established by FESS ethmoidectomy, reserving external ethmoidectomy for failures.
    e. Adenoidectomy may improve the outlook in chronic maxillary sinusitis.

46. *Synopsis 239–240; Scott-Brown 4/12/14–24*
a. False FESS may be effective and avoid the need for external
operation. The ethmoid is almost always infected
anyway. There is, however, a risk that FESS in this
area may result in subsequent stenosis, making
drainage worse and risking late mucocoele formation.
b. False The Lynch-Howarth procedure comprises fronto-
ethmoidectomy via a curved incision around the
medial border of the orbit. Patterson's approach,
where the incision is below the orbital margin, is used for
combined access to maxillary and ethmoidal sinuses.
c. True   The objective is to form a wide drainage channel from
the frontal and anterior ethmoidal cells into the
middle meatus.
d. True   This is usually performed only after failure of more
conservative measures.
e. False It is hinged inferiorly.

47. *Synopsis 243–245; Scott-Brown 4/12/25–26, 6/17/9–14*
a. False Antibody deficiency is a rare cause.
b. True.
c. False Cultures are usually mixed in chronic cases. *H.
influenzae* is often responsible for acute sinusitis.
d. True.
e. False Kartagener's syndrome consists of sinusitis, bronchiectasis
and dextrocardia. The common defect is in ciliary
structure. The fact that the kinocilium is affected
results in loss of polarity in embryonic development
and, hence, dextrocardia. The heart condition is
asymptomatic; this is a favourite of examiners!

48. *Synopsis 243–245; Scott-Brown 4/12/25–26, 6/17/9–14*
a. True   Frontal sinusitis is therefore rare in infants.
b. True.
c. False Pain is often absent. Nasal obstruction, mucopurulent
rhinorrhoea, mouth breathing, snoring, coughing and
ear problems are the main clinical features. Early
morning vomiting may occur.
d. False Conservative management is preferred. Predisposing
factors such as allergy should be treated, and
neighbouring infections controlled.
e. True   Chronically infected and enlarged adenoids act as a
source of infection and may obstruct normal drainage,
which is via the nasopharynx.

49. **Spread of infection in suppurative sinusitis:**
    a. Osteitis occurs in compact bone.
    b. Osteomyelitis occurs in diploic bone.
    c. Meningitis usually arises via a septic thrombophlebitis.
    d. Lymphatic channels are involved in the formation of subperiosteal abscesses.
    e. Spread into the subarachnoid space can occur via the perineural space around the olfactory nerves.

50. **Osteomyelitis of the frontal bone:**
    a. This is most frequently due to frontal sinusitis.
    b. Streptococci and staphylococci are the commonest bacteria responsible.
    c. The onset is usually acute, with rigors or epileptic fits.
    d. 'Pott's puffy tumour' is a malignant myxomatous degeneration.
    e. Intracranial complications are a remote possibility.

51. **Osteomyelitis of the frontal bone:**
    a. X-rays do not show any bony abnormality until sequestration occurs.
    b. Antibiotic treatment is ineffective.
    c. The floor of the frontal sinus should be trephined in severe cases with sequestration and intracranial infection.
    d. Opening the anterior wall of the sinus is contraindicated.
    e. Where bone has to be removed in young patients, the defect may regenerate spontaneously.

49. *Synopsis 245–246; Scott-Brown 4/13/1–2*
a. True.
b. True.
c. True   Further spread causes intracranial venous sinus thrombosis, and extradural, subdural and brain abscesses. Distant venous spread may cause septicaemia and endocarditis.
d. True   The lymphatics accompany blood vessels through their bony foramina.
e. True.

50. *Synopsis 246; Scott-Brown 4/13/8*
a. True   It occurs particularly where the sinus is operated on without antibiotic cover.
b. True   The streptococci may be anaerobic.
c. False   The onset is usually insidious, with dull local pain. Rigors and fits occur later, signifying septicaemia and intracranial spread respectively.
d. False   Pott's puffy tumour is an oedematous swelling of the soft tissues overlying the infected bone.
e. False   An extradural abscess is likely to follow unless treatment is prompt.

51. *Synopsis 246; Scott-Brown 4/13/8*
a. False   In the first week there will be no changes other than those of the frontal sinusitis or trauma. A loss of bone pattern then appears, followed by thinning, necrosis and sequestration.
b. False   High-dose intravenous antibiotics are the mainstay of treatment.
c. False   This procedure would be inadequate for such cases. They would require more radical surgery.
d. False   The anterior wall of the sinus must be opened where sequestration has occurred, to remove the dead and infected bone.
e. True   However, grafts will often be necessary.

52. **Orbital complications of suppurative sinusitis:**
    a. All the paranasal sinuses border the orbit at some point.
    b. Orbital complications are most common in children.
    c. Preseptal cellulitis is associated with severe pain and proptosis of the globe.
    d. Orbital cellulitis usually precedes abscess formation.
    e. Thrombophlebitis may result in cavernous sinus thrombosis.

53. **Orbital complications of suppurative sinusitis:**
    a. Loss of colour vision is a late sign of visual loss.
    b. Proptosis means that an abscess has formed.
    c. The fundus in orbital cellulitis is pale because of compression of the ophthalmic artery.
    d. A CT scan is mandatory if vision is deteriorating rapidly.
    e. A rapidly growing orbital tumour can simulate orbital cellulitis.

54. **Intracranial complications of suppurative sinusitis:**
    a. The frontal sinus is the commonest source of a brain abscess.
    b. Ethmoidal sinusitis is associated with diffuse suppurative meningitis.
    c. Sphenoidal sinusitis is associated with cavernous sinus thrombosis.
    d. Papilloedema, nausea, vomiting and decreased consciousness are early signs of an extradural abscess.
    e. A subdural empyema is best treated by multiple burr holes.

52. *Synopsis 247–248; Scott-Brown 4/13/3–6, 4/24/3–5*
 a. True   However, most clinical cases are due to spread of infection from the ethmoids.
 b. True   Orbital complications are usually due to ethmoidal infection.
 c. False   Preseptal cellulitis is the least severe form, with non-tender oedema restricted to the eyelids, no oedema within the orbit and no displacement of the globe or visual impairment.
 d. True   Progession may be rapid.
 e. True.

53. *Synopsis 247–248; Scott-Brown 4/13/3–6, 4/24/3–5*
 a. False   Loss of colour vision is an early warning sign, which usually occurs before any loss of visual acuity.
 b. False   Proptosis simply means that the globe has been displaced forward. Any expanding mass in the orbit can do this.
 c. False   The fundus shows congestion because of venous compression.
 d. False   Emergency surgical decompression is required. Unless the scan can be done immediately, without signficantly delaying surgery, it should be omitted.
 e. True.

54. *Synopsis 248, 545–560; Scott-Brown 4/13/6–8*
 a. True   Extradural and subdural abscesses and thrombophlebitis of the sagittal sinus and cortical veins over the frontal lobe may also occur.
 b. True   The route of spread is usually via the roof of the ethmoidal labyrinth.
 c. True   It is also associated with diffuse meningitis and with thrombophlebitis of other intracranial venous sinuses.
 d. False   The early signs may be subtle – a persistent headache, fever and general malaise – and easily confused with symptoms of the underlying sinusitis.
 e. False   A subdural empyema will require formal craniotomy as well as treatment of the underlying sinusitis and prolonged intravenous antibiotics.

55. **Secondary effects of suppurative sinusitis:**
    a. Infection from the nasopharynx may cause laryngitis.
    b. Sinus infection may cause chronic secretory otitis media.
    c. Chronic maxillary sinusitis causes bronchiectasis.
    d. Treatment of sinusitis should precede thoracic surgery where sinusitis and bronchiectasis coexist.
    e. Successful treatment of chronic sinusitis may improve asthma.

56. **Transitional cell papillomas (Ringertz tumours):**
    a. These are indistinguishable from simple inflammatory nasal polyps on rhinoscopy.
    b. Most arise from the nasal septum.
    c. They may have areas of columnar and squamous epithelium.
    d. Malignant transformation only occurs after irradiation.
    e. Complete removal is the treatment of choice.

55. *Synopsis 249; Scott-Brown 4/15/9–14, 5/4/10, 5/5/1–9, 6/7/3–6*
a. True   A chronic postnasal drip of infected mucopus may cause lateral pharyngitis, tonsillitis and laryngitis.
b. True   Streams of mucopus may be seen in the region of the Eustachian tube orifice on endoscopic examination of the nasopharynx.
c. False The two conditions are associated and exacerbate one another, but the relationship is not causal. Some rare cases are due to a congenital defect in ciliary motility (Kartagener's syndrome) or to abnormally viscid mucous secretion (cystic fibrosis); others may be due to the long-term effects of damage to the respiratory tract sustained during a childhood attack of pertussis or measles.
d. True   Sometimes medical treatment with topical steroids will suffice, otherwise sinus surgery is indicated.
e. True   Such treatment can sometimes allow the dose of steroids and bronchodilators to be reduced.

56. *Synopsis 249–250; Scott-Brown 4/3/12–13, 5/23/22–23*
a. False Most will be unilateral, whereas inflammatory polyps are usually bilateral. The surface appearance is different, being grey and wrinkled or fleshy rather than the gelatinous appearance of a typical polyp. However, no gross appearance is diagnostic, and cases will be missed unless all polyps are sent for histology.
b. False The majority arise from the lateral nasal wall, some from the antrum or ethmoidal sinuses.
c. True   The epithelium is grossly thickened and infolded, leading to the alternative pathological description of 'inverted papilloma'. Epithelial atypia is common, but the basement membrane remains intact.
d. False There is an incidence of around 5 per cent malignancy; there is dispute as to whether this is malignant transformation or whether the malignant tumours are malignant from the outset. Malignant behaviour may be early or delayed many years. Radiotherapy should not be used prophylactically for non-malignant cases.
e. True   This can sometimes be achieved endoscopically; otherwise a lateral rhinotomy or midfacial degloving approach is required.

57. **Benign tumours of the paranasal sinuses:**
    a. Ivory osteoma of the frontal sinus is the commonest type.
    b. The commonest presentation is headache due to pressure erosion of the anterior cranial fossa.
    c. Mucocoele and ocular displacement are complications of frontal sinus osteoma.
    d. Localized fibro-osseous dysplasia in children should be excised completely because of the danger of malignant change.
    e. Torus palatinus usually requires excision.

58. **Malignant tumours of the nose and paranasal sinuses:**
    a. Squamous cell carcinoma is the commonest type.
    b. Retropharyngeal and cervical lymph node metastases are common.
    c. Adenoid cystic carcinoma is associated with woodworkers in the furniture industry.
    d. An ameloblastoma is a rapidly growing, highly malignant tumour.
    e. Burkitt's lymphoma is confined to African children.

The nose and sinuses

57. *Synopsis 250–252; Scott-Brown 4/3/13–15, 4/22/7, 4/24/13–14, 6/16/34–38*
    a. True   Incidence: up to 1 per cent of skulls.
    b. False The commonest presentation is an incidental finding on X-ray.
    c. True   These occur when the tumour obstructs the fronto-nasal duct or is large enough to expand into the orbit.
    d. False Malignant change is not a problem unless the condition is unwisely treated with radiotherapy. A biopsy may be necessary to differentiate the dysplasia from a malignant tumour, but following this it is best left alone until growth has ceased, when cosmetic reduction can be undertaken. Earlier surgical intervention may be necessary if local complications ensue, such as a threat to vision from orbital involvement.
    e. False This midline exostosis of the hard palate is usually an incidental finding and requires no treatment. It may need to be removed if it interferes with the fitting of dentures.

58. *Synopsis 252–257; Scott-Brown 5/23/21–36*
    a. True   80 per cent of malignant tumours are of this type. The majority of them are poorly differentiated.
    b. False Metastases occur in about 5 per cent of cases. Failure to control local disease is the usual cause of death.
    c. False Adenocarcinoma is associated with woodworkers in the furniture industry.
    d. False It is slowly growing and relatively benign.
    e. False Cases have occurred elsewhere, including the USA, and in adults as well as children.

59. Malignant tumours of the paranasal sinuses:
   a. CT or MRI scanning is essential to determine the extent of the tumour.
   b. Bantu tribesmen in South Africa who burn mahogany, and wood machinists in the hardwood furniture industry, share a high risk of upper jaw cancer.
   c. Pain is the earliest clinical feature.
   d. Epiphora indicates an antral primary.
   e. Biopsy is usually unnecessary as the diagnosis can be made radiologically.

60. Treatment of malignant tumours of the paranasal sinuses:
   a. Surgery should be reserved for cases where there is a good prospect of cure.
   b. If the tumour penetrates the cribriform plate it is inoperable.
   c. Radical surgery followed by radiotherapy gives 5-year survival figures of 80 per cent overall.
   d. Orbital involvement is a contraindication to radical maxillectomy.
   e. Cytotoxic drug treatment is the first line of management.

59. *Synopsis 252–257; Scott-Brown 5/23/21–36*
a. True   Plain X-rays are inadequate. CT is best for displaying bone erosion, but does not differentiate well between tumour and secondary inflammation and retained secretions; MRI gives better soft tissue differentiation. Therefore, both methods should be employed.
b. True   Interestingly, the Bantu tend to get squamous carcinoma whereas the woodworkers get adenocarcinoma of the nose and sinuses.
c. False   Pain is usually late, from involvement of the maxillary nerve, facial tissues or dura.
d. False   Epiphora is due to nasolacrimal duct or sac obstruction. This is most commonly due to fronto-ethmoidal tumours, although an antral tumour can spread into this area. In practice it is often difficult to specify the exact site of origin, as the tumours tend to be quite extensive at presentation.
e. False   Biopsy is essential. It may be carried out via the nose, endoscopically, or via an antrostomy. The Caldwell-Luc operation was previously recommended for antral tumours, but is now unnecessary with modern endoscopic techniques and it risks seeding tumour into the facial tissues.

60. *Synopsis 255–256; Scott-Brown 5/23/25–36*
a. False   The condition is naturally mutilating, and death may be delayed and unpleasant. Surgery can offer palliation with an improvement in quality of life even where cure is not possible.
b. False   Craniofacial resection gives good results, provided the brain has not been invaded.
c. False   The 5-year survival rate is unlikely to exceed 50 per cent.
d. False   Orbital clearance is combined with radical maxillectomy in such cases.
e. False   Cytotoxic chemotherapy is still confined to the role of adjuvant treatment. It is potentially dangerous, and should only be carried out in specialized hospital units – preferably as part of a controlled trial, since further information on efficacy is still required.

√ **61. Pituitary tumours:**
    a. Most pituitary tumours are malignant.
√   b. Acromegaly is usually due to an acidophil adenoma.
    c. Cushing's syndrome can be treated by hypophysectomy.
    d. Transphenoidal hypophysectomy is particularly suitable for suprasellar tumours.
    e. The optic chiasma is at greater risk from transfrontal craniotomy than from a transphenoidal approach.

62. Maxillary cysts:
    a. A midline swelling in the palate is likely to be malignant.
    b. A median alveolar cyst is of developmental origin.
    c. A nasopalatine cyst arises from the incisive canal, and can present either in the nose or on the palate.
    d. A lateral alveolar cyst separates incisor from canine teeth, at the line of fusion between maxilla and premaxilla.
√   e. A naso-alveolar cyst usually presents as a loose tooth.

63. Cysts of dental origin:
    a. Primordial cysts are malignant.
    b. A cyst of eruption arises over a tooth that has not erupted.
    c. A tooth is usually inside a dentigerous (follicular) cyst.
    d. Dental (radicular) cysts imply previous or current root infection.
    e. A dental cyst may persist after root extraction.

64. Radiographic diagnosis of maxillary cysts:
    a. A clear outline is typical of developmental cysts.
    b. Multiple cysts may be due to cherubism.
    c. Hyperparathyroidism characteristically causes a single giant cyst with a sharply defined margin.
    d. An osteoclastoma is usually radiolucent.
    e. A myelomatous deposit is usually radio-opaque.

61. *Synopsis 256–257; Scott-Brown 4/23/1–10*
  a. False Nearly all pituitary tumours are benign.
  b. True Modern cytohistochemical methods stain according to the hormone produced. Acromegalics produce excessive growth hormone.
  c. True Cushing's syndrome can be treated by hypophysectomy, provided it is due to an ACTH-secreting pituitary tumour rather than an adrenal tumour or a side effect of steroid therapy.
  d. False A small suprasellar extension is not a contraindication, but large suprasellar lesions will need a craniotomy.
  e. True.

62. *Synopsis 257–261; Scott-Brown 4/22/1–9, 5/23/1–18*
  a. False It is likely to be of developmental origin.
  b. True It lies between the upper central incisors.
  c. True.
  d. True.
  e. False It usually presents as nasal obstruction, or external deformity with a wide nostril and loss of the nasolabial fold. It lies in the floor of the nose anteriorly and displaces the inferior turbinate upwards.

63. *Synopsis 257–261; Scott-Brown 4/22/1–9, 5/23/1–18*
  a. False A primordial cyst is formed from enamel organ epithelium before dental tissue.
  b. True.
  c. True.
  d. True.
  e. True.

64. *Synopsis 257–261; Scott-Brown 4/22/1–9, 5/23/1–18*
  a. True.
  b. True The cysts are symmetrically arranged, affecting both maxilla and mandible.
  c. False It causes multiple poorly-defined radiolucent areas, with alteration of normal bony trabeculation.
  d. True.
  e. False It is radiolucent with a round 'punched out' appearance.

√ 65. Odontogenic tumours:
a. Odontogenic tumours arise solely from developing dental epithelium.
b. They are commonest in young adults and children.
c. An adamantinoma contains enamel.
d. A composite odontoma is so called because it incorporates more than one tooth.
e. An ameloblastoma is likely to metastasize widely.

66. Causes of epistaxis:
a. Idiopathic bleeding from Little's area is commonest.
b. Digital trauma (nose-picking) is a common cause.
c. A septal spur predisposes.
d. Low atmospheric pressure and low humidity increase the incidence.
e. Venous hypertension is a factor in chronic bronchitics.

67. Sites of bleeding in epistaxis:
a. Little's area is the anterior end of the inferior turbinate.
b. Kiesselbach's plexus is in the pterygopalatine fossa.
c. Bilateral epistaxis implies bleeding from the nasopharynx.
d. Bleeding above the level of the middle turbinate is likely to originate from the internal carotid artery.
e. Bleeding from the middle meatus may be due to a tumour in the maxillary sinus.

65. *Synopsis 257–261; Scott-Brown 4/22/1–9, 5/23/1–18*
a. False   They may also arise from mesodermal elements.
b. True.
c. False   Now known as ameloblastoma, this locally invasive
tumour probably arises from the epithelial debris of
Malassez, which comprises remnants of the primary
dental lamina.
d. False   A composite odontoma is so called because it is
formed of more than one germinal layer – ectoderm
and mesoderm.
e. False   It is locally malignant (cf. basal cell carcinoma).

66. *Synopsis 261–265; Scott-Brown 4/18/1–17*
a. True.
b. True.
c. True   This also makes treatment difficult. Septal surgery may
be required.
d. True   Both factors operate together at altitude.
e. True.

67. *Synopsis 261–265; Scott-Brown 4/18/1–17*
a. False   Little's area is the anterior part of the septum.
b. False   Kiesselbach's plexus is in Little's area.
c. False   Bilateral epistaxis is commonly due to the original side
being partially blocked by the patient or by clot; blood
then passes behind the choana and down the opposite
nasal fossa. Alternatively, there may be more than one
site, but bleeding from the nasopharynx is rare.
d. True   Bleeding is likely to be from the anterior ethmoidal, a
branch of the ophthalmic, supplied from the internal
carotid artery.
e. True   This is a rare cause.

68. Management of severe epistaxis:

    a. The patient should be placed head-down and supine, with a pillow under the shoulders.

    b. The use of cocaine 5 per cent nasal spray is contraindicated because of the risk of worsening hypertension.

    c. It is preferable to cauterize any accessible bleeding points rather than immediately packing the nose.

    d. A postnasal pack should be considered when the haemoglobin falls below 10 g/l.

    e. A central venous pressure line is mandatory.

The nose and sinuses

68. *Synopsis 263–265; Scott-Brown 4/18/9–14*

a. False It is difficult to think of a worse position. The patient should be seated in a chair, leaning forward, breathing through the open mouth, and allowing blood to drip into a bowl. The anterior part of the nose is compressed between finger and thumb to put pressure on Little's area, which is the site of bleeding in 90 per cent of cases. Ice packs can be applied to the forehead or bridge of the nose. An atmosphere of calm efficiency should prevail.

b. False Cocaine should be sprayed into the nasal fossae for its vasoconstrictor and local anaesthetic properties, which may then allow cautery or packing to be performed with better vision and less discomfort to the patient.

c. True The use of a rigid or flexible fibreoptic endoscope may help in localizing the source of bleeding, though it is not always possible to cauterize a site more posteriorly, particularly if it is beyond a septal deviation.

d. False A postnasal pack is used when an adequate anterior pack fails to control bleeding. A haemoglobin of 10 g/l is not compatible with life (=1 g/dl).

e. False This is rarely required unless complications are present.

69. **Surgical intervention in epistaxis:**
    a. Failure to control bleeding by cautery or packing for 48 hours is an indication for surgical intervention.
    ✓ b. Submucous resection is indicated only for gross septal deformities where it is impossible to pass a rigid nasal endoscope.
    c. Endoscopic or transantral ligation of the maxillary artery is ineffective because of collateral circulation from the circle of Willis.
    d. Ligation of the common carotid is a useful alternative to maxillary ligation in the elderly patient.
    e. The anterior ethmoidal artery can be approached via a Howarth incision.

70. **Epistaxis in hereditary haemorrhagic telangiectasia:**
    a. This is rarely a significant problem.
    ✓ b. Androgens are used in treatment.
    c. Injection of sclerosants is usually curative.
    d. Septodermoplasty involves excision of the septal mucosa and replacing it with a split skin graft.
    e. Bleeding may occur lower down the gastrointestinal tract.

69. *Synopsis 264–265; Scott-Brown 4/18/14–16*
   a. True   Although opinions vary as to how long conservative measures should be tried, there is good evidence that if bleeding has not been controlled by 48 hours of nasal packing, the overall hospital stay is reduced by surgical intervention at that stage.
   b. False   Submucous resection may be beneficial even in relatively minor deformities if access is improved. It may have an additional mode of action by interrupting the blood supply to Little's area and the haemorrhagic nodules, and could therefore be of benefit even when the septum is entirely straight.
   c. False   Maxillary artery ligation is usually an effective operation. Failure is due to technical deficiency, collateral circulation from the opposite side or bleeding from the anterior ethmoidal artery.
   d. False   Ligation of the common carotid would probably cause a stroke or death of the patient. External carotid ligation is occasionally useful, as it is quick and can be performed under local anaesthetic if necessary. The problem of collateral circulation is less if it is tied distal to the lingual branch.
   e. True.

70. *Synopsis 265; Scott-Brown 4/18/16–17*
   a. False   Bleeding is frequent, and can be severe. No treatment is permanently effective; multiple blood transfusions and operations are often required.
   b. False   Oestrogens are used in treatment.
   c. False.
   d. True   This will be effective for 2–3 years, after which telangiectases recur on the grafted area.
   e. True   This can be fatal, despite control of nosebleeds.

71. **Intrinsic (vasomotor) rhinitis:**
    a. The nasal mucosa is hyper-reactive.
    b. Parasympathetic over-activity is implicated.
    c. Puberty may initiate the condition.
    d. Symptoms are usually worse in pregnancy.
    e. Rhinitis medicamentosa is due to beta blockers.

72. **Clinical features of intrinsic (vasomotor) rhinitis include the following:**
    a. Paroxysmal sneezing attacks.
    b. Alternating intermittent bilateral nasal obstruction.
    c. Thick, green, foul-smelling rhinorrhoea.
    d. Nasal polyps.
    e. Mulberry turbinates.

73. **Medical treatment of intrinsic (vasomotor) rhinitis:**
    a. Precipitating factors should be identified and avoided if possible.
    b. Antihistamines are especially useful for obstructive symptoms.
    c. Topical steroids are the mainstay of medical treatment.
    d. Vasoconstrictors should be administered systemically.
    e. Epistaxis is a recognized side effect of topical steroids.

71. *Synopsis 265–267; Scott-Brown 4/9/1–15*
  a. True   A wide range of trigger factors cause excessive secretion, sneezing and vasodilatation, by non-allergic mechanisms.
  b. True.
  c. True   This is presumably due to an endocrine effect.
  d. True.
  e. False   Beta blockers do cause nasal congestion in some patients, but rhinitis medicamentosa refers to chronic hypertrophic rhinitis with rebound congestion caused by excessive prolonged use of local sympathomimetic vasoconstrictor drops.

72. *Synopsis 265–267; Scott-Brown 4/9/1–15*
  a. True   These are easily confused with allergic reactions.
  b. True   Obstruction is often positional, with the dependent nostril becoming blocked while lying on the side in bed.
  c. False   This would suggest sinus infection or a foreign body.
  d. True   Polyps are particularly likely in the sub-group of intrinsic rhinitis characterized by eosinophilia in the nasal secretions.
  e. True   Their name refers to a bulky, polypoidal appearance of the posterior ends of the inferior turbinates.

73. *Synopsis 265–267; Scott-Brown 4/9/1–15*
  a. True   Smoking and alcohol especially should be avoided.
  b. False   They are sometimes useful for sneezing and profuse watery rhinorrhoea.
  c. True   Administration is either by spray or drops.
  d. False   This can be dangerous; tachyphylaxis occurs, limiting usefulness.
  e. True   A different formulation may help.

74. Surgical treatment of intrinsic (vasomotor) rhinitis:
  a. Surgery is necessary in the majority of cases.
  b. Nasal obstruction associated with hypertrophy of the inferior turbinates and failure to respond to topical nasal steroids is the principal indication for submucosal diathermy.
  c. Septal surgery may be helpful, even if the cartilaginous deformity is minor.
  d. Radical reduction of the inferior turbinates is ineffective and dangerous, and should no longer be performed.
  e. For a long-term cure, Vidian neurectomy is the procedure of choice.

75. Aetiology of allergic rhinitis:
  a. It is often familial.
  b. IgE is the reaginic antibody.
  c. Coexisting asthma or eczema implies atopy.
  d. Inhaled allergens are the commonest trigger factor.
  e. Aspirin gives relief by reducing the inflammatory reaction.

74. *Synopsis 265–267; Scott-Brown 4/9/1–15*
a. False   The majority can be managed medically. Local steroids
           have been a great advance.
b. True   Diathermy to the inferior turbinates, either surface or
           submucosal, is used to reduce their bulk to help relieve
           nasal obstruction. However, this tends to be of only
           temporary benefit, with the obstruction often recurring
           after 12–18 months.
c. True   What appears as a minor deformity can be significant
           in the context of intermittent mucosal swelling.
d. False   The operation is effective, but can cause severe
           primary or reactionary haemorrhage in 1–2 per cent of
           cases. It should be performed as an inpatient.
e. False   Vidian neurectomy offers an apparently logical
           approach to the autonomic imbalance and is usually
           effective initially, but in most hands the symptoms
           recur after 2–3 years and the operation has now lost
           favour. The long-term results are poor.

75. *Synopsis 268; Scott-Brown 4/6/2–4*
a. True   This is probably through multifactorial genetic
           influences.
b. True   It is formed in the nasal mucosa following contact with
           the allergen, and causes release of vasoactive and
           inflammatory mediators from mast cells.
c. True   Atopy is an exaggerated IgE antibody response to
           aero-allergens, which results in a predisposition to
           developing allergic diseases such as rhinitis, asthma
           and eczema.
d. True   The commonest allergen is house dust mite faeces.
           Ingested allergens may also play a role, and there are
           numerous non- specific additional triggers such as
           exercise, sudden temperature change and
           psychological upset.
e. False   Aspirin is itself a potent trigger factor, especially in
           atopic patients with asthma.

76. **Immunology of allergic rhinitis:**
    a. Most patients have a specific allergy to one substance only.
    b. IgE is released by the mast cells.
    c. There is a Type I hypersensitivity reaction.
    d. Histamine leaks from the endothelial cells via loosened desmosomal junctions.
    e. IgG is involved in some cases.

77. **Pathology of allergic rhinitis:**
    a. Oedematous swelling of the mucosa is due to plasma leakage from loosened junctions between capillary endothelial cells.
    b. There is infiltration with giant epithelioid cells.
    c. Seromucinous glands atrophy.
    d. Venous stasis results in a dusky swelling of the inferior turbinates.
    ✓ e. Polyp formation is a rare complication.

78. **Clinical features of allergic rhinitis:**
    a. Symptoms may be seasonal or perennial.
    b. Age of onset is usually in the fourth decade.
    c. Anosmia is the main complaint.
    d. Sneezing attacks may be incapacitating.
    e. Polyps should be suspected if nasal obstruction is permanent.

79. **Treatment of allergic rhinitis:**
    a. Avoidance of allergens is frequently impractical.
    b. Desensitization based on skin testing is useful in some cases of hay fever.
    c. Vasoconstrictor drops provide effective immediate relief.
    d. Antihistamines give useful relief of nasal obstruction, but have little effect on sneezing and rhinorrhoea.
    e. Topical steroids and sodium cromoglycate both act to reduce the hypersensitivity reaction.

76. *Synopsis 268; Scott-Brown 1/18/17, 4/6/4–8*
  a. False Multiple allergies are the rule; hence the poor success
             rate of allergen avoidance and desensitization.
  b. False IgE is released by modified B lymphocytes, plasma cells.
             It binds to the mast cells causing them to degranulate,
             releasing histamine, 5-hydroxytryptamine, tryptase,
             bradykinin, prostaglandins and leukotrienes, which
             modulate an acute inflammatory reaction.
  c. True.
  d. False Histamine is released from mast cells. The tight junctions
             between the endothelial cells do leak plasma, causing oedema.
  e. True IgG_4 is involved, with a Coombs and Gell Type III reaction.

77. *Synopsis 269–270; Scott-Brown 4/6/4–8*
  a. True.
  b. False Eosinophils and plasma cells predominate. Giant
             epithelioid cells are a histological feature of tuberculosis.
  c. False They are hyperactive.
  d. True.
  e. False Polyps are common in both allergic and non-allergic rhinitis.

78. *Synopsis 270–271; Scott-Brown 4/6/8–9*
  a. True.
  b. False Onset is usually in childhood or early adult life.
  c. False Sneezing, running and blocked nose are the main
             complaints. Anosmia does occur.
  d. True.
  e. True   In uncomplicated allergy, the nasal obstruction is
             intermittent.

79. *Synopsis 271–272; Scott-Brown 4/6/10–14*
  a. True   This is particularly so where multiple allergies are present.
  b. True   This is now carried out much less frequently in the
             UK, since national guidelines were issued on the
             necessity for full cardiopulmonary resuscitation
             facilities in case of anaphylactic reaction.
  c. True   They are therefore very popular. The problem is that
             prolonged use leads to rhinitis medicamentosa.
  d. False The opposite is true.
  e. True.

80. **Surgical treatment of allergic rhinitis:**
    a. This is preferable to long-term medication in children.
    b. Surgery is indicated where chronic nasal obstruction is due to polyps.
    c. Adenoidectomy is the first line of treatment in children.
    d. Reduction of the inferior turbinates is indicated for sneezing.
    e. Vidian neurectomy can be performed by a transantral approach.

81. **Pathology of nasal polyps:**
    a. Simple inflammatory polyps are usually bilateral.
    b. Epithelial metaplasia occurs in polyps associated with non-allergic eosinophilic rhinitis.
    c. Infective maxillary sinusitis may exacerbate nasal polyposis.
    d. Malignant polyps are usually clinically indistinguishable from benign ones.
    e. Childhood nasal glioma is a malignant polyp.

82. **Antrochoanal polyps:**
    a. These are commonest in the elderly.
    b. They are usually multiple.
    c. Unilateral nasal obstruction is the commonest symptom.
    d. The maxillary sinus is opaque on X-ray.
    e. Most can be completely removed intranasally.

The nose and sinuses

80. *Synopsis 272; Scott-Brown 4/9/12–14, 4/10/10–12, 6/17/11–12*
a. False   Surgery is an adjunct rather than an alternative to medical treatment. No operation will cure the underlying allergic tendency.
b. True.
c. False   Allergic rhinitis is not an indication for adenoidectomy.
d. False   Antihistamines are indicated for chronically hypertrophic turbinates causing nasal obstruction. The operation has little or no effect on sneezing or rhinorrhoea.
e. True.

81. *Synopsis 272–273; Scott-Brown 4/10/1–9*
a. True   Therefore, a unilateral polyp should provoke suspicion of more sinister aetiology.
b. True   There is a progression from columnar to squamous. This may occur in any inflammatory polyp.
c. True   Infected mucus may cause further inflammatory reaction and swelling of the oedematous polyp tissue.
d. False   Malignant polyps are usually unilateral; they may bleed or produce bloody discharge, and cause pain or other local symptoms. Surface appearance varies; they may be ulcerated or fleshy, but this is not typical of the benign mucosal variety. Cervical metastases may be present.
e. False   It is a benign tumour, possibly a hamartoma rather than a true neoplasm.

82. *Synopsis 273–276; Scott-Brown 4/10/14*
a. False   They are most common in adolescents and young adults.
b. False   Antrochoanal polyps are usually found singly.
c. True.
d. True.
e. False   A Caldwell-Luc approach is often required, although endoscopically assisted intranasal polypectomy should be tried first. It is helpful when attempting intranasal removal to aspirate fluid via an antral puncture, deflating the antral part of the polyp so that it can be teased out via the ostium. The use of a 70°-angled rigid nasal endoscope helps visualize the antral portion of the polyp via the natural ostium, which is usually much larger than normal.

83. **Treatment of simple nasal polyps:**
    a. Betamethasone nasal drops will shrink some polyps.
    b. Systemic steroids are occasionally used in severe cases.
    c. Antihistamines may improve rhinorrhoea and sneezing.
    d. Simple snaring of polyps is no longer performed because of the high incidence of recurrence.
    e. Functional endoscopic ethmoidectomy is the initial treatment of choice.

84. **Epiphora:**
    a. This is excessive watering of the eye due to nasolacrimal duct or sac obstruction.
    b. Congenital atresia is the commonest cause.
    c. It may be due to a malignant tumour of the maxillary antrum.
    d. Initial treatment is by probe and syringe.
    e. Dacrocystorhinostomy aims to divert tears to the opposite nostril via a plastic tube passed through the septum.

83. *Synopsis 274–276; Scott-Brown 4/10/10–14, 4/12/17–24*
a. True   They will shrink up to 50 per cent of polyps. Surgery
can sometimes be avoided.
b. True   However, they are unsuitable for prolonged treatment.
c. True   This is particularly so when polyps are associated with
rhinitis.
d. False   Although eventual recurrence is common, the procedure
is effective and relatively safe. Post-operative local
steroid treatment is advised in recurrent cases.
e. False   Topical steroids should be used first. Until recently, most
UK surgeons regarded intranasal ethmoidectomy
(endoscopic or otherwise) as intrinsically dangerous, and
would advocate repeated simple polypectomy, reserving
external ethmoidectomy for severe cases. Endoscopic
techniques have proved as safe as other methods in
experienced hands.

84. *Synopsis 276–277; Scott-Brown 4/12/24–25, 4/24/9–10, 5/23/24*
a. True.
b. False   Chronic dacrocystitis is the commonest cause.
c. True   Sinus X-rays should be performed routinely.
d. True   This is the province of the ophthalmologist.
e. False   Tears are directed to the same side. The sac is opened
and sewn to the lateral nasal wall proximal to the site
of obstruction.

The larynx and tracheobronchial tree

1. **Development of the larynx:**
   a. The tracheobronchial groove appears cephalic to the hypobranchial eminence.
   b. The thyroid cartilage develops from the fourth arch cartilage.
   ✓ c. The superior laryngeal nerve is the branchial nerve of the sixth arch.
   ✓ d. The sixth arch artery persists on the left.
   e. The early embryonic position of the larynx is high up under the tongue.

2. **The infantile larynx in comparison with the adult:**
   a. The infantile larynx is the same relative size as the adult larynx.
   b. It has its narrowest point in the supraglottis.
   c. It lies at a higher level than the adult larynx.
   d. It collapses easily due to the lack of muscular support.
   e. It has an inlet lying less oblique.

3. **Cartilaginous framework of the larynx:**
   a. The thyroid alae meet to make an angle of 120° in the female.
   b. Calcification of the posterior part of the cricoid lamina can be confused radiographically with a foreign body.
   c. The epiglottis is formed of elastic fibrocartilage.
   d. The cartilages of Wrisberg do not articulate with any other.
   ✓ e. The crico-arytenoid joint can both rotate and glide.

1. *Synopsis 417; Scott-Brown 1/12/1–2*
   a. False It is caudal to the hypobranchial eminence. The tracheobronchial is also called the laryngotracheal groove.
   b. True.
   c. False The superior laryngeal nerve supplies the fourth branchial arch; the recurrent laryngeal is the nerve of the sixth arch.
   d. True This persists as the ductus arteriosus in the neonate, and as the ligamentum arteriosum in the adult. Due to its persistence the left recurrent laryngeal nerve courses through the thorax.
   e. True With maturation it assumes a position lower down; in the adult it is usually opposite C6/7.

2. *Synopsis 419; Scott-Brown 1/12/3–4*
   a. False It is relatively and absolutely smaller.
   b. False It is narrowest at the subglottis; hence any further constriction by disease rapidly leads to respiratory embarrassment.
   c. True It is virtually under the tongue at birth. It descends during growth to lie opposite C6/7 in the adult.
   d. False It collapses easily because the laryngeal cartilages are softer than in the adult. On forced inspiration they tend to collapse more easily.
   e. True This plane of the laryngeal inlet means a greater risk of aspiration.

3. *Synopsis 419; Scott-Brown 1/12/3–4*
   a. True In men it is about 90°; hence the pronounced 'Adam's apple' in males.
   b. True.
   c. True.
   d. True These are also called cuneiform cartilages, and are contained within the mucosa of the aryepiglottic fold.
   e. True Rotation moves the vocal process medially or laterally, and gliding adducts or abducts the arytenoids.

4. **Laryngeal musculature:**
   a. Only the posterior crico-arytenoid muscle abducts the vocal cords.
   ✓ b. All the intrinsic muscles are paired.
   c. The inferior constrictor steadies the larynx during phonation.
   ✓ d. The vocalis consists of the lower and deeper fibres of thyro-arytenoid.
   e. Contraction of the thyrohyoid can either lower the hyoid or raise the larynx.

5. **In the cavity of the larynx:**
   a. The rima glottidis is the interval between the false cords.
   b. Reinke's space is found between the surface epithelium and the deeper elastic layer.
   c. Keratinizing stratified squamous epithelium lines the true cords.
   ✓ d. The posterior part of the ventricular sinus contains the mucus-secreting saccule.
   e. The length of the glottis is about 1.6 cm in the adult female.

6. **Neurovascular supply and lymphatic drainage of the larynx:**
   a. The main blood supply is from branches of the superior and inferior thyroid arteries.
   b. Lymph from the supraglottic larynx drains to the pre-epiglottic and upper deep cervical nodes.
   c. The internal branch of the superior laryngeal nerve is entirely motor.
   d. The external branch of the superior laryngeal nerve supplies the cricothyroid muscle.
   e. The recurrent laryngeal nerve is sensory above the true cords.

4. *Synopsis 424–425; Scott-Brown 1/12/8–10*
   a. True   This paired muscle is the sole abductor.
   b. False They are all paired except for the transverse arytenoid, or interarytenoid, muscle.
   c. False Although attached to the larynx, it has no effect on its movement.
   d. True   This is also called the internal tensor of the vocal cords, the external tensor being the cricothyroid muscle.
   e. True   If the hyoid is fixed the larynx is raised and vice versa.

5. *Synopsis 426–427; Scott-Brown 1/12/7–8*
   a. False It is between the true cords and has an anterior intermembraneous part and a posterior intercartilaginous section.
   b. True   This is a large potential space in the true cords, which may fill with fluid leading to Reinke's oedema.
   c. False It is non-keratinizing.
   d. False The saccule is located in the anterior part of the sinus. Its secretion constantly lubricates the vocal cords.
   e. True   It is about 2.5 cm in the adult male.

6. *Synopsis 427–428; Scott-Brown 1/12/44*
   a. True.
   b. True.
   c. False It is entirely sensory down to the level of the true cords.
   d. True.
   e. False It is sensory below the vocal cords.

7. **Physical examination of the larynx:**
   a. The anterior commissure is easily visualized on indirect laryngoscopy during quiet inspiration.
   b. The use of a 70°- or 90°-Hopkins rod telescope allows 80 per cent of larynges to be visualized.
   c. Stroboscopy is of most value in studying vocal cords during quiet respiration.
   d. Antero-posterior tomography is valuable in assessing the degree of subglottic carcinoma.
   e. MR is poorer at demonstrating metastatic nodal disease than clinical examination.

8. **Protective functions of the larynx:**
   a. The aryepiglottic sphincter closes during deglutition and vomiting.
   b. The false cord sphincter is primarily involved in preventing ingress of foreign material.
   c. The true vocal cords have a curved inferior surface with the concavity directed inferiorly.
   d. The false cord sphincter cannot be closed independently of the true vocal cords.
   e. The cough reflex consists of four phases.

9. **During deglutition:**
   a. Only the aryepiglottic sphincter closes.
   b. The larynx is lowered to assist passage of the food bolus into the pharyngo-oesophageal opening.
   c. Laryngeal airflow continues in an outward direction.
   d. The epiglottis tilts forwards.
   e. The apposed true vocal cord sphincter can resist a pharyngeal pressure of 150 mmHg.

7. *Synopsis 429; Scott-Brown 5/1/3–4, 5/2/5–8, 5/2/13*
   a. False   It is usually only visualized on vocalization of the sound 'e'.
   b. True   This figure includes both adult and paediatric patients.
   c. False   Stroboscopy gives a slow motion view of the vocal cords during phonation. It is particularly useful in the study of speech physiology and in the analysis of abnormal voice production.
   d. True   However, both CT and MR scanning are superior as they allow accurate assessment of soft tissue and skeletal structures.
   e. False   Both MR and CT are superior to clinical examination.

8. *Synopsis 436–438; Scott-Brown 1/11/2, 1/13/10*
   a. True   Its action opposes the aryepiglottic folds. Anteriorly the closure is completed by the epiglottic tubercle, and posteriorly by the bodies of the arytenoid cartilages. The epiglottis per se is not essential in preventing aspiration and it can be surgically removed without complications.
   b. False   It acts as a mechanical flap valve, due to its anatomical shape, preventing egress of air. It helps produce the rise in intratracheal pressure needed for coughing, sneezing, micturition and parturition. It offers little resistance to the ingress of air, but is useful in preventing aspiration of foreign material by physiological muscular contraction.
   c. True   This shape offers minimal resistance to air outflow, and resists pressure from above.
   d. True.
   e. True   The four phases are inspiration, compression, expiration and cessation.

9. *Synopsis 315; Scott-Brown 1/11/2, 6*
   a. False   All three sphincters (aryepiglottic, false cord and true cord) undergo reflex contraction during the pharyngeal phase.
   b. False   It is elevated to bring about this situation.
   c. False   Airflow ceases completely during deglutition.
   d. False   The epiglottis tilts backwards to help deflect the food into the pyriform fossae.
   e. True   This, combined with the 30 mmHg resistance offered by the false cords to tracheal pressure, minimizes the risk of aspiration during deglutition.

10. **In voice production:**
    a. The frequency of tone can be altered by adjusting the shape of the free margin of the vocal cords.
    b. Articulation is performed by the vibrating cords.
    c. Infraglottic air pressure changes do not alter pitch.
    d. The vocal folds are lengthened by the action of the cricothyroid muscle.
    e. The volume of sound produced is governed by the infraglottic pressure.

11. **Symptoms and signs of laryngeal disease in the newborn include the following:**
    a. Failure to thrive.
    b. Cough.
    c. Tracheal plunging.
    d. Croup.
    e. Tachycardia.

12. **Congenital laryngeal stridor (laryngomalacia):**
    a. The laryngeal superstructure is soft and may be oedematous.
    b. The epiglottis is normal.
    c. Presentation may be failure to thrive.
    d. Amputation of the epiglottis is effective treatment.
    e. The condition usually resolves, without treatment, between the second and fifth years of life.

10. *Synopsis 437; Scott-Brown 1/12/11–12, 5/6/4–7*
   a. True   This occurs as the voice registers are changed. The edges
           are thick in low registers and thin in higher ones. This
           alteration is produced by contraction of the deep fibres
           of the thyro-arytenoid (vocalis) muscle.
   b. False The vocal cords phonate – i.e. produce the basic sound
           of the voice – at a pitch determined by their frequency
           of vibration. Timbre is added by the resonating
           structures of the vocal tract (pharynx, oral cavity, nose
           etc.). Articulation is the breaking up of the sound into
           recognizable language phonemes by the coordinated
           action of the palate, tongue, jaws and lips.
   c. False An increase in infraglottic air pressure leads to a rise
           in intensity and a slight increase in pitch.
   d. True   It increases the antero-posterior dimensions of the
           laryngeal inlet and hence lengthens the vocal folds.
   e. True   The greater the infraglottic pressure, the louder the
           volume. The intensity is also proportional to the area
           of mouth opening.

11. *Synopsis 442–443; Scott-Brown 6/22/2–3*
   a. True   Breathing and feeding difficulties are usually
           associated in these cases.
   b. True   This is particularly so if there is an irritative lesion in
           the larynx or there is overspill into the
           tracheobronchial tree.
   c. True   A high negative pressure in the pleural cavity sucks the
           larynx and trachea into the thorax.
   d. True   Croup is the same as inspiratory stridor.
   e. True   This is an almost invariable accompaniment of
           laryngeal disease.

12. *Synopsis 442–443; Scott-Brown 6/22/1–2*
   a. True.
   b. False It is usually elongated, thin and folded on itself – the
           so-called 'omega' shape.
   c. True   The commonest symptom, however, is inspiratory
           stridor. The stridor is diminished by rest and made
           worse by exertion or upper respiratory tract infection.
   d. False.
   e. True   However, there is a small risk of death from
           respiratory infection, especially in the first year of life.

13. **Congenital laryngeal web:**
    a. Symptoms may be absent.
    b. This usually involves the posterior one-sixth of the vocal cords.
    c. The voice is of normal quality.
    d. Excision should be performed as early as possible.
    e. A complete atresia may be the cause of stillbirth.

14. **In compression (closed) injuries of the larynx:**
    a. Submucosal haemorrhage may result in marked dyspnoea and hoarseness, with minimal external signs.
    b. The cricoid cartilage is most frequently fractured.
    c. A fixed vocal cord means that the recurrent laryngeal nerve has been damaged.
    √ d. If there is any doubt regarding the airway, an immediate tracheostomy should be performed.
    e. Perichondritis may be prevented by performing urgent tracheostomy.

15. **Laryngeal trauma:**
    a. In inhalation burns, oedema of the vocal cords is the commonest finding.
    b. Heimlich's manoeuvre may be effective in expelling an inhaled foreign body
    c. The use of relaxant drugs has increased the incidence of intubation injuries.
    √ d. Flat foreign bodies in the larynx tend to lie antero-posteriorly in the long axis of the larynx.
    e. Laryngectomy may be necessary for a radiotherapy reaction.

13. *Synopsis 444; Scott-Brown 6/22/23*
 a. True Symptoms may be absent if the web is small.
 b. False It usually involves the anterior one-sixth. The fusion may extend inferiorly to the upper margin of the cricoid cartilage.
 c. False Hoarseness is an invariable symptom.
 d. False Most cases do not need treatment. Thin webs can be divided endoscopically, using normal microlaryngeal instruments or laser. Insertion of a keel, either endoscopically or via a laryngofissure approach, will usually be necessary for thicker webs. A tracheostomy may be required for severe stridor or dyspnoea, but excision via a laryngofissure should be delayed until the larynx is mature.
 e. True This is also easily overlooked at autopsy.

14. *Synopsis 445–446; Scott-Brown 5/8/1–10*
 a. True.
 b. False Hyoid and thyroid cartilage fractures are much more common. Cricoid fractures are likely to be fatal.
 c. False Damage to the recurrent laryngeal nerve is one cause of a fixed cord, but it may be due to traumatic dislocation of the crico-arytenoid joint or to post-traumatic fibrosis.
 d. False Endotracheal intubation is preferable in the first instance.
 e. False Perichondritis may be prevented by administering prophylactic systemic antibiotics and debridement as indicated.

15. *Synopsis 447–449, 468–469; Scott-Brown 5/1/10, 5/11/2–3,14,23–25*
 a. False Usually only the supraglottis is involved, the vocal cords being spared.
 b. True Heimlich's manoeuvre is a sudden 'bear hug' from behind, with the arms encircling the patient just below the xiphisternum.
 c. False The use of relaxant drugs has reduced the incidence of intubation injuries. Intubation injuries are due to traumatic insertion, an oversized tube, an over-inflated cuff, excessive tube movement or prolonged intubation.
 d. True They may therefore not be seen on antero-posterior radiographic views. Flat foreign bodies in the pharynx lie in a transverse plane, and may not be seen on a lateral view. Hence, always insist on both AP and lateral views.
 e. True This is particularly so in severe intractable cases with respiratory embarrassment and lack of voice. Also, severe reactions may mask the continuing presence or recurrence of tumour.

16. **Abnormal voice production:**
    a. Functional mutational voice disorders are common.
    b. Whispering psychogenic aphonia is commoner in women.
    c. Contact ulcers occur as a result of abnormal approximation of the vocal processes of the arytenoid.
    d. Weightlifting may produce acute submucosal haemorrhage on the vocal cords.
    e. Most voice failures in singers are due to inadequate training.

17. **Acute simple laryngitis in children:**
    a. This may be associated with exanthemata.
    b. Stridor is more likely to occur than in adult acute laryngitis.
    c. Gastro-oesophageal reflux may have an aetiological role.
    d. This must be distinguished from an inhaled foreign body.
    e. An oxygen/helium mixture may be beneficial.

18. **Acute epiglottitis:**
    a. Inflammatory changes affect mainly the submucosa of the sinus of Morgagni.
    b. Pharyngeal symptoms predominate in the adult.
    c. X-rays should be performed.
    d. The causal organism is usually a corynebacterium.
    e. Systemic steroids are essential.

16. *Synopsis 450, 461, 484–485; Scott-Brown 5/5/10, 5/6/12–13, 5/11/3–4*
a. False   These are rare. If the male is shaving and has acne and a prominent 'Adam's apple', androgenic activity is likely to be normal. Intersex and eunochoidism is very rare.
b. True   This is usually a reaction to stress, and is a conversion symptom.
c. True   They are commonest in adult males who persistently abuse the voice, e.g. street vendors. Gastro-oesophageal reflux may be an aetiological factor. Biopsy should be carried out to exclude cancer, though occurrence of cancer at this site, the vocal process, is very rare.
d. True   This is due to the violent and forced closure of the vocal cords, necessary to raise the intrathoracic pressure and splint the diaphragm.
e. True.

17. *Synopsis 454; Scott-Brown 5/5/1–2, 6/24/6*
a. True.
b. True.
c. True.
d. True   The absence of a raised temperature or other signs of infection should alert the doctor to the possibility of a foreign body.
e. True   Heliox (helium 80 per cent, oxygen 20 per cent) has a much lower density than air, reducing the resistance to flow through a compromised laryngeal inlet.

18. *Synopsis 455; Scott-Brown 5/5/1–2, 6/24/8–11*
a. False   They affect mainly the loosely attached mucosa of the epiglottis.
b. True   In a child, laryngeal rather than pharyngeal symptoms are manifest.
c. False   X-rays are usually difficult in a terrified child, and this delays treatment.
d. False   The causal organism is usually *Haemophilus influenzae* type B. Most cases are in children aged 3–4 years. The disease is much less common in the UK since the introduction of vaccination against *H. influenzae*.
e. False   Intravenous antibiotics are necessary. Although commonly administered, the value of steroids has never been proven.

19. **Acute laryngotracheobronchitis:**
    a. This is associated with influenza epidemics.
    b. It produces copious volumes of serous exudate.
    c. A relatively quiet chest on auscultation is a good prognostic sign.
    d. It must be distinguished from diphtheria.
    e. It can lead to rapid overhydration if untreated.

20. **Hyperkeratosis of the larynx:**
    a. This should be treated with radiotherapy.
    b. It produces impairment of cord mobility.
    c. It gives a nibbled appearance, due to ulceration of the free cord margin.
    d. It is characterized by a 'washleather' ulceration of the epiglottis.
    e. This is a precancerous condition.

19. *Synopsis 456; Scott-Brown 5/5/2–3*
   a. True   It is initiated by a virus, usually parainfluenza type I.
                Bacterial infection, particularly with the haemolytic
                streptococcus or *Staphylococcus aureus* may
                occasionally supervene, causing a very severe illness.
   b. False Secretions are thick, tenacious, difficult to expel, and
                occur throughout the respiratory tract.
   c. False A quiet or silent chest is a sign of imminent respiratory
                failure. Atelectasis is common due to the obstruction
                of small bronchi.
   d. True   Differentiation is by bacteriological examination.
                Removal of a diphtheritic membrane causes
                underlying mucosal bleeding.
   e. False Dehydration is very common, and must be prevented
                by intravenous fluid supplements if indicated.

20. *Synopsis 460–461; Scott-Brown 5/11/14*
   a. False Repeated stripping of the cords is the usual practice
                unless frank carcinoma supervenes.
   b. False.
  ✓ c. False This appearance is characteristic of tuberculous
                laryngitis.
  ✓ d. False This appearance is seen in the tertiary form of
                acquired syphilis, and represents the gummatous
                lesion.
   e. True   There is a significant risk of progression to carcinoma
                in situ and frank invasive carcinoma. These patients,
                predominantly men, should be kept under regular review.

21. **Recurrent respiratory papillomatosis:**
    a. This commonly involves the vocal cords and ventricular bands.
    b. It is primarily a disease of young adults.
    c. It should be treated with radiotherapy.
    d. Laryngectomy may be required.
    e. It is caused by a haemolytic positive streptococcus.

22. **Benign lesions of the larynx:**
    a. Vocal cord polyps comprise localized oedema in Reinke's space.
    b. Mucus retention cysts occur most commonly in the ventricular sinus.
    c. Chondromata usually arise from the arytenoid cartilages.
    d. Laryngeal amyloidosis is usually subglottic, and presents with increasing stridor.
    e. A laryngocoele is an air-containing prolongation of the laryngeal ventricle.

23. **In the 1987 UICC classification of carcinoma of the larynx:**
    a. The posterior commissure is part of the glottis.
    b. A glottic tumour involving both cords with normal mobility and no extension to other sites is a T1b lesion.
    c. A tumour limited to the larynx with cord fixation is T3.
    d. The presence of two cervical lymph node metastases makes the patient Stage IV.
    e. A thyroid cartilage chondrosarcoma that has invaded into the thyroid gland is T4.

21. *Synopsis 470; Scott-Brown 6/34/1–5*
a. True   It may spread to the epiglottis, trachea and bronchi.
b. False   Infants and young children are mostly affected, but it may continue into adult life.
c. False   This mode of treatment can lead to damage of laryngeal cartilages, and there is a risk of malignant change in the long term. Repeated endoscopic removal of the papillomata, with conservation of normal structures, is required. Suction diathermy has been superseded by CO_2 laser for this purpose.
d. True   Laryngectomy may be required in severe cases of the disease, or if stenosis due to scarring occurs. Tracheostomy is sometimes necessary, but should be avoided if possible because further spread can occur into the tracheobronchial tree and, occasionally, into the parenchyma of the lungs.
e. False   It is probably caused by the human papilloma virus (HPV) types 6 and 11. Genital warts in the mother at the time of delivery increase the risk of offspring developing the disease in early childhood.

22. *Synopsis 470–471, 477–478; Scott-Brown 5/6/14–15, 5/11/1–6, 6/22/2–4, 6/34/1–5*
a. True.
b. False   They occur most commonly in the supraglottis, on or adjacent to the epiglottis, and are often asymptomatic. Infection causes enlargement, and may be a cause of stridor. They are usually treated by endoscopic removal.
c. False   These are uncommon tumours that arise in the subglottis, frequently the posterior plate of the cricoid cartilage.
d. False   This is usually supraglottic, the commonest site being the ventricular bands. Symptoms vary according to the site. Subglottic amyloid does cause increasing stridor.
e. True.

23. *Synopsis 474; Scott-Brown 5/11/11,19–21,42–43*
a. True.
b. True   'b' is for both cords, 'a' is for a single cord.
c. True.
d. True   Nodal metastasis is one of the major prognostic factors. Any distant metastasis also makes the patient stage IV, as does local spread of the primary beyond the larynx (T4) even without nodal or distant metastasis.
e. False   The classification only applies to squamous carcinoma.

24. **Spread of malignant disease of the larynx:**
    a. Tumours of the anterior commissure can extend directly into the petiolus.
    b. The true vocal cords are virtually devoid of lymph vessels.
    c. About 40 per cent of tumours of the false cords and ventricular sinuses have metastasized at the time of diagnosis.
    d. There is a lack of transglottic lymph vessels in a vertical direction.
    e. Otalgia suggests cartilage invasion.

25. **Total laryngectomy:**
    a. This may be useful as a palliative measure in locally advanced malignancy.
    b. The Sorenson U-flap incision may be unsatisfactory after high-dose radiotherapy.
    c. Continuous sutures in the inferior constrictor muscle should be avoided in the repair of the pharyngeal wall.
    d. A long posterior pharyngeal myotomy improves the chances of achieving good speech with a Blom-Singer valve.
    e. Prophylactic use of antibiotics active against anaerobes has helped to reduce the incidence of post-operative pharyngocutaneous fistula.

24. *Synopsis 472–473; Scott-Brown 5/11/16–22*
a. True This usually occurs at an early stage. They can also invade the thyroid cartilage. Anterior commisure lesions have a poor prognosis.
b. True This explains the more favourable prognosis and the basis of limited local excision such as cordectomy.
c. True This is because of the later presentation and the abundant lymphatics, which crossflow, making contralateral and bilateral nodal pathology very likely.
d. True This is the pathophysiological basis of a partial supraglottic laryngectomy. Transglottic tumours are likely to be due to direct growth in both directions rather than a consequence of lymphatic spread.
e. True This usually occurs with perichondritis.

25. *Synopsis 475; Scott-Brown 5/11/26–37*
a. True This may be the most reliable method of controlling and relieving distress due to a fungating lesion.
b. True The tip may necrose. However, it is frequently employed because it has the advantages of good exposure and easier suturing around the tracheostome, and skin incisions are distant from the pharyngeal repair sutures.
c. False The pharyngeal defect should be sutured in two layers. The first should be a continuous extramucosal inverting suture layer (Connell suture) including the inferior constrictor; the second interrupted layer is a reinforcement, and should cover the first.
d. True.
e. True Good surgical technique, haemostasis and an adequately prepared and nourished patient have also helped to reduce the incidence of this problem.

26. **Laryngocoeles:**
    a. These are caused by dilatation of the subglottis.
    b. The external variety project through the thyrohyoid membrane.
    c. They can easily be demonstrated with plain X-rays.
    d. Early excision is advisable.
    e. They may be caused by tumour.

27. **Oedema of the larynx:**
    a. The glottis is the site most frequently affected.
    b. The oedema may be caused by an idiosyncratic reaction to iodine.
    c. This is a complication of Ludwig's angina.
    d. 0.5 ml of 1:1000 adrenaline should be given intramuscularly in an adult.
    e. Stertorous breathing implies subglottic oedema.

28. **Episodes of stridor:**
    a. Expiratory stridor usually indicates supraglottic obstruction.
    b. An inhaled foreign body should be excluded.
    c. A vocal cord paralysis may be present.
    d. If due to laryngomalacia, the prognosis is good.
    e. In an infant with a normal appearance of the larynx, an enlarged thymus may exist.

26. *Synopsis 477; Scott-Brown 5/16/17–18*
a. False   Laryngocoeles are caused by dilatation of the ventricle and saccule of the larynx.
b. True   The internal laryngocoele resembles a cyst underneath the ventricular band. Up to 50 per cent are combined internal and external laryngocoeles.
c. True   This is particularly so during a forced Valsalva manoeuvre.
d. False   This is only advisable if symptoms of hoarseness or dyspnoea are troublesome. The internal laryngocoele can be uncapped endoscopically, and the external variety by an external approach that may include division of the thyroid cartilage.
e. True   This is especially the case with lesions in the ventricle, which may create a valve effect. Neoplasia should be excluded in all cases by direct laryngoscopy.

27. *Synopsis 478–480; Scott-Brown 5/5/5, 6/21/1, 6/24/1–16*
a. False   Oedema occurs in areas where the mucosa is loosely adherent, i.c. the supraglottis (vestibule and aryepiglottic folds) in adults and the subglottis in children. Acute epiglottitis is potentially lethal in children.
b. True   This is an allergic phenomenon producing rapid anaphylaxis (angioneurotic oedema). Aspirin and certain food substances are also potential allergens.
c. True   Ludwig's angina is a rapidly progressive brawny swelling of the submandibular region and floor of mouth due to bacterial infection, and is often secondary to dental sepsis.
d. False   It should be given subcutaneously. In a child, an initial dose of 0.1 ml is sufficient. Systemic steroids are also indicated. Breathing Heliox (helium 80 per cent, oxygen 20 per cent) may be helpful.
e. False   Stertor implies airway obstruction above the level of the laryngeal inlet. Biphasic stridor is characteristic of subglottic obstruction.

28. *Synopsis 442–443, 454–457, 478–484; Scott-Brown 6/21/1–9*
a. False   Expiratory stridor or wheeze indicates bronchial obstruction, commonly due to asthma. Supraglottic obstruction causes inspiratory stridor.
b. True.
c. True   Both unilateral and bilateral recurrent laryngeal nerve palsies may produce intermittent symptoms.
d. True   Most children will improve spontaneously with age.
e. True.

29. **Neural paralysis of the larynx:**
    a. Aspiration is more likely if the superior laryngeal nerve is affected.
    b. The paralysed cord usually lies at a lower level.
    c. If due to bronchial carcinoma, the primary pathology is easily diagnosed in most cases.
    d. In bilateral abductor paralysis, the patient has a good voice but is subject to stridor.
    e. The retention of an efficient cough reflex and lack of aspiration in apparent bilateral adductor paralysis implies non-organic disturbance (hysterical aphonia).

30. **Management of laryngeal paralysis:**
    a. Surgical treatment of idiopathic unilateral recurrent laryngeal nerve paralysis should be delayed for 9–12 months to allow for spontaneous recovery.
    b. Paralysis due to mediastinal spread from carcinoma of the oesophagus indicates a possibility of surgical cure.
    c. Laser arytenoidectomy is particularly useful in unilateral lesions.
    d. Cordopexy obviates the need for a tracheostomy in bilateral recurrent nerve lesions.
    e. Teflon paste injection for unilateral paralysis is of little value.

31. **Voice disorders:**
    ✓ a. Phonaesthenia (myasthenia of the larynx) is usually due to neurological disease.
    b. Video-stroboscopic laryngoscopy improves visualization of the medial vibrating surfaces of the vocal folds compared with conventional laryngoscopy.
    c. Vocal nodules are caused by habitual dysphonia, and require surgical removal for cure.
    d. Dysphonia plicae ventricularis (ventricular band voice) may be caused by compensatory efforts in vocal disabilities.
    e. Virilization of the voice in women caused by androgenic anabolic steroids is easily reversible on stopping the drugs.

29. *Synopsis 482–487; Scott-Brown 5/5/15–16, 5/9/12–15*
  a. True   There is loss of sensation in the supraglottis.
  b. True.
  c. True   This is usually obvious on the chest X-ray. However, in rare cases a left recurrent nerve paralysis may appear before there is any evidence of lung carcinoma.
  d. True.
  e. True.

30. *Synopsis 482–485; Scott-Brown 5/9/11–19*
  a. True   In the interim, voice therapy aimed at strengthening the opposite adductor may be employed.
  b. False This indicates inoperability. The same is true of bronchial carcinoma.
  c. False It may be employed in bilateral abductor paralysis. The airway can be improved, but usually at the expense of the voice. In many cases, a tracheostomy with speaking valve is preferable.
  d. True   This is its only advantage. The voice quality is usually poor.
  e. False This is a very valuable procedure, and is the treatment of choice for adductor paralysis in recurrent nerve lesions due to carcinoma of the lung, oesophagus and breast.

31. *Synopsis 484–485; Scott-Brown 5/6/11*
  a. False It is usually due to vocal misuse or laryngitis. Myasthenia gravis and myotonia atrophica are rare neurological causes.
  b. True   It may therefore be possible to see minor irregularities, which are blurred during a conventional view on phonation.
  c. False Nodules can disappear within weeks with voice rest. Re-education of the voice is the treatment of choice.
  d. True   It may be caused particularly by compensation in myasthenia. False cord opposition produces an extremely rough voice.
  e. False The size of the vocal folds increases, and this is usually irreversible.

32. Development of the trachea and bronchi:
   a. The rudimentary respiratory tree appears during the third or fourth week of embryonic life as a median laryngotracheal groove in the ventral wall of the pharynx.
   b. A congenital tracheo-oesophageal fistula is due to failure or arrest of formation of the tracheo-oesophageal septum.
   ✓c. The lung bud forms three lobules on the left side.
   d. The non-respiratory bronchiolar division is complete by birth.
   ✓ e. The number of alveoli does not increase after birth.

✓ **33. Anatomy of the trachea:**
   a. The manubrio-sternal angle is an external landmark for the carina.
   b. The normal full-term neonatal trachea is 5–6 mm in internal diameter.
   ✓ c. The diameter of the trachea is greater during expiration than inspiration.
   d. The mucosal lining is transitional ciliated columnar epithelium.
   e. The recurrent laryngeal nerve supplies the trachea.

34. Relations of the trachea in the neck:
   a. The recurrent laryngeal nerves lie in the groove between the trachea and the vertebral bodies.
   b. The thymus lies behind the trachea.
   c. The thyroid isthmus is at a higher level in children than adults.
   d. Lymphatic drainage is to the deep cervical nodes.
   e. The recurrent laryngeal nerves pass in front of the inferior thyroid artery.

32. *Synopsis 491; Scott-Brown 1/12/1–3, 6/22/4–5*
  a. True   The groove deepens, then its edges fuse to form a tube from which the larynx, trachea and bronchial tree develop.
  b. True.
  c. False There are three on the right and two on the left.
  d. True.
  e. False Alveoli continue to increase in number until the age of 8 years, then increase in size until chest wall growth is complete.

33. *Synopsis 491–493; Scott-Brown 1/12/18–19, 6/25/3–4, 6/26/2*
  a. True   This is at the second costal cartilage. The precise position is dependent on posture and the respiratory cycle.
  b. True.
  c. False The diameter increases during inspiration. In the bronchi, this may allow easier passage of forceps for removal of a foreign body.
  d. False The lining is pseudostratified ciliated columnar epithelium with an abundance of goblet cells.
  e. True   The recurrent nerve is both motor and sensory to the trachea.

34. *Synopsis 492; Scott-Brown 1/12/18–24, 1/18/14–15*
  a. False It lies in the groove between the trachea and the oesophagus.
  b. False It is anterior to the trachea at the root of the neck, and is larger in children than adults.
  c. True   In adults it usually crosses the second, third and fourth tracheal rings.
  d. False Drainage is to the pre- and paratracheal nodes.
  e. False The nerves can be in front, behind or amongst the terminal branches of the inferior thyroid artery.

35. In the tracheobronchial tree:
   a. A bronchopulmonary segment consists of a segment of lung with its segmental bronchus.
   b. Aspiration in a supine patient is most likely to cause problems in the apical bronchus of the right lower lobe.
   c. The left brachiocephalic vein lies anterior to the thoracic trachea in the adult.
   d. Respiratory bronchioles are supported by complete rings of cartilage.
   e. The carina is 25 cm from the incisor teeth in the average adult.

36. In the upper air passages:
   a. The length of cervical trachea can alter in any one individual.
   b. The trachea is nearest to the skin at the fourth tracheal ring.
   c. The larynx descends during postnatal growth.
   d. The pleural dome is at risk during tracheostomy.
   e. The cricoid cartilage may be more easily palpated than the thyroid cartilage.

37. In performing a tracheostomy:
   a. The head should be extended to a maximum degree.
   b. A vertical tracheal incision should be avoided in children.
   c. The tracheal incision should always include the first tracheal ring.
   d. The tracheostomy tube should fit tightly without a cuff.
   e. Tapes should be tied with the head in the neutral position.

35. *Synopsis 493–497; Scott-Brown 1/12/26–28*
a. True.
b. True   This is a frequent site of pneumonitis, collapse or abscess formation.
c. True   However, it may project superiorly and hence be in danger during tracheostomy. In infants, the brachiocephalic artery may produce similar complications because of its higher position.
d. False   Cartilage support in the tracheobronchial system occurs only as far as bronchioles of 1 mm in diameter.
e. True   This is a useful landmark when an orotracheal tube is inserted.

36. *Synopsis 492–493; Scott-Brown 1/12/26–28, 6/25/3–4, 6/26/2*
a. True   This varies with physique and degree of neck extension.
b. False   The trachea is nearest to the skin immediately below the cricoid cartilage.
c. True   It descends from C3 in the infant to about C6 in the adult.
d. True   The contents of the mediastinum may enter the neck when the latter is extended, in particular the pleural domes and left brachiocephalic vein. In infants, the thymus and brachiocephalic artery may be involved.
e. True   This is particularly so in infants, as the definitive configuration of the thyroid cartilage takes place at puberty.

37. *Synopsis 498–503; Scott-Brown 1/12/26–27, 5/7/8–18, 6/26/4–7*
a. False   Such a manoeuvre may lead to both the skin incision and tracheal fenestration being placed too low. If this occurs in an adult, post-operative nursing may be difficult; in a neonate, the stoma may end up behind the manubrium. Additionally, there is the risk of drawing up mediastinal contents into the neck during the procedure (e.g. brachiocephalic vessels).
b. False   It is the most suitable incision, giving the least risk of transection. In the long term, it also results in less stenosis and airways resistance.
c. False   This predisposes to subglottic stenosis.
d. False   The tube should be a loose fit.
e. False   The head should be slightly flexed.

38. **In the post-operative care of tracheostomy:**
    a. Constant nursing attention, with humidification, and suction of secretions as required, should be provided for at least 24 hours.
    b. Post-operative lateral cervical and chest X-rays should be performed in children.
    c. Copious mucus production indicates a pulmonary infection.
    d. A poorly positioned tracheostomy tube may produce a fatal haemorrhage.
    e. Mucus and crusts are the commonest causes of obstruction.

39. **In a child with a tracheostomy:**
    a. Endoscopy prior to decannulation is useful rather than essential.
    b. There may be a predisposition to recurrent chest infections.
    c. Stomal granulations rarely occur if proper nursing care is given.
    d. Surgical decannulation may result in surgical emphysema.
    e. Fatal tube obstruction or accidental decannulation is most likely to occur in the early hospitalized period.

38. *Synopsis 501–503; Scott-Brown 1/12/26–27, 5/7/11–12, 6/26/7–10*
a. True.
b. True   These will indicate whether the tracheostomy tube is correctly sited. In children, a tube that is too long and lodged in the right main bronchus can be demonstrated.
c. False   The tracheobronchial secretions increase in volume, and this is a normal reaction. It does not indicate infection, but this may supervene if regular suction is not performed or if the mucus dries and a crust obstructs the lung, causing atelectasis.
d. True   A tracheostomy tube tip may erode the anterior tracheal wall and the brachiocephalic artery.
e. True   Others include a prolapsed cuff or an infant's chin.

39. *Synopsis 501–503; Scott-Brown 6/26/7–10, 6/27/1–7*
a. False   Endoscopy is essential. It allows assessment of the suprastomal region for granulations, subglottic narrowing, tracheal wall collapse and vocal cord movements.
b. True   The child may benefit from a trial of decannulation.
c. False   Stomal granulations occur in nearly all cases, despite best efforts.
d. True   This is particularly so if the tracheal stoma is inadequately sutured.
e. False   This is most likely to occur as a late complication, at home.

MCQs in Otolaryngology

40. Congenital abnormalities of the tracheobronchial tree:
    a. These account for less than 5 per cent of cases of congenital stridor.
    b. They include bulging of the posterior tracheal wall.
    c. Narrowing due to tracheomalacia is worse during expiration
    d. Posterior tracheal compression is usually due to an aberrant left subclavian artery.
    e. Vascular compression of the trachea with severe symptoms is best managed by tracheostomy.

41. Acquired subglottic stenosis:
    a. Excessive movement of an endotracheal tube is a cause.
    b. The pathology includes perichondritis of the cricoid.
    c. Repeated dilatation is the treatment of choice.
    d. Mild cases present as stridor following an upper respiratory tract infection.
    e. Early laryngotracheal reconstruction with cartilage grafting may avoid the need for tracheostomy.

42. Tracheobronchial foreign bodies:
    a. These are most common between the ages of 10 and 15 years.
    b. They are characterized by an initial episode of choking.
    c. They may present as a unilateral wheeze.
    d. They can cause a haemoptysis.
    e. They become symptomatic within a few days.

40. *Synopsis 505–506; Scott-Brown 6/22/4–7*
   a. False   Congenital abnormalities account for about 25 per
                  cent of cases of congenital stridor.
   b. False   This is a normal finding in neonates due to laxity of the
                  trachealis.
   c. True   The localized form is due to external compression. The
                  less common generalized tracheomalacia usually
                  recovers spontaneously, although occasionally
                  insertion of a long tracheostomy tube is required.
   d. False   An aberrant right subclavian artery passes between the
                  trachea and oesophagus, and produces symptoms
                  referable to one or both structures. An aberrant left
                  subclavian artery compresses the oesophagus alone as
                  it passes posterior to it.
   e. False   Tracheostomy should be avoided. Bypassing the
                  obstruction may result in intubation of the right main
                  bronchus, and there is a risk of erosion of the artery by
                  the tube tip. Patients with significant symptoms should
                  have a surgical decompression via thoracotomy.

41. *Synopsis 468–469; Scott-Brown 6/22/3–4, 6/23/1–7*
   a. True   This causes mucosal abrasion and ulceration.
   b. True   The perichondritis is followed by chondritis,
                  granulations and fibrosis.
   c. False   Dilatation may help in selected cases of congenital
                  subglottic stenosis.
   d. True   A history of neonatal intubation should also be sought.
   e. True.

42. *Synopsis 506–508; Scott-Brown 6/25/1–10*
   a. False   Most inhaled foreign bodies occur in children below
                  4 years of age.
   b. False   Tracheobronchial foreign bodies are characterized
                  usually by paroxysmal coughing.
   c. True   In a child without a history of asthma, this symptom
                  should lead to a search for an inhaled foreign body.
   d. True   Vegetable matter in particular causes a florid mucosal
                  reaction with marked granulations.
   e. False   After the initial bout of coughing, symptoms may cease.
                  This may be the case for several months if the foreign body
                  is an inert substance producing little mucosal reaction.

43. Management of an inhaled foreign body:
a. Unilateral emphysema and mediastinal shift on a chest X-ray indicate complete obstruction of a bronchus.
b. Conservative management with bronchodilators, postural drainage and thoracic percussion should be employed initially.
c. Adrenaline 1:1000 should be instilled into the forceps space.
d. The Clerf-Arrowsmith forceps are useful for removing peanuts.
e. Systemic steroids should be administered if the procedure was prolonged.

44. Inflammatory processes in the tracheobronchial tree:
a. Tracheitis sicca may be improved by laryngectomy.
b. Dextrocardia may rarely be present.
c. Acute laryngotracheobronchitis is more common in boys.
d. Antitoxins are not required if tracheal diphtheria is treated with systemic penicillin.
e. Foreign bodies should always be excluded.

43. *Synopsis 506–508; Scott-Brown 5/1/10–13, 6/25/2–10*
a. False This indicates a partial obstruction with valvular effect.
Air is able to enter on inspiration, when the air
passages dilate slightly, but on expiration the bronchus
is blocked by contraction onto the foreign body.
Complete obstruction causes atelectasis, and may be
followed by a lung abscess.
b. False The value of these measures is very limited, and there
is a danger of the foreign body impacting in the
subglottis. Rigid endoscopy and removal under general
anaesthetic by a skilled team is the treatment of
choice.
c. False Topical adrenaline or cocaine is useful on granulations
to reduce bleeding, and may shrink some mucosal
oedema by its vasoconstrictor action. The forceps
space is the gap that usually exists between an
irregularly-shaped foreign body and the bronchial wall.
It may enlarge during inspiration and close during
expiration.
d. False These forceps are used for the removal of safety pins.
e. True Steroids are indicated if the procedure is prolonged or
if there is a risk of subglottic oedema, particularly in
children.

44. *Synopsis 456, 508–510; Scott-Brown 5/5/2–3, 5/7/16, 5/11/33,
6/24/4–6*
a. False Tracheitis sicca may be caused by laryngectomy. It is
occasionally associated with atrophic rhinitis and
laryngitis sicca. The dry crusts require humidification
to soften them and, occasionally, formal toilet to
remove them.
b. True This is known as Kartagener's syndrome –
bronchiectasis, chronic sinusitis and dextrocardia.
c. True It is especially common in boys under 4 years of age,
and is most frequently caused by parainfluenza virus
type I.
d. False Antitoxins are essential to neutralize the endotoxins
that can produce myocarditis and peripheral neuritis.
e. True They should particularly be excluded in children, and
in those with recurrent problems or unilateral signs.

45. Carcinoma of the bronchus:
   a. A persistent unproductive cough is an early symptom.
   b. Hoarseness due to involvement of the left recurrent laryngeal nerve means there has been hilar invasion.
   c. Ptosis is associated with paralysis of the hand.
   d. Dysphonia caused by cord palsy should be treated with a course of speech therapy.
   e. It may present as an enlarging cervical node.

46. Tracheal stenosis:
   a. Tracheomalacia is the commonest cause.
   b. Simple excision of up to 8 cm length of trachea with end-to-end anastomosis is possible.
   c. The recurrent laryngeal nerve is at greater risk from repeated dilatations than from excision of the stenosis.
   d. Grillo and Barclay described a procedure involving detachment of the right main bronchus from the bifurcation and its reattachment distally to the left main bronchus.
   e. Thyroidectomy is contraindicated if a goitre is causing external compression.

45. *Synopsis 514–517; Scott-Brown 5/9/13–17*
   a. True   The cough later becomes productive of purulent and
              bloodstained sputum.
   b. False   Hilar invasion may cause recurrent laryngeal nerve
              paralysis, but an apical tumour may compromise either
              recurrent nerve and cause similar symptoms. The
              nerve may also be involved by metastases in the neck.
   c. True   An apical tumour (Pancoast's) invades the brachial
              plexus (causing shoulder pain and hand paralysis) and
              the cervical sympathetic chain (causing Horner's
              syndrome – ptosis, meiosis, enophthalmos and loss of
              facial sweating).
   d. False   Improvement with speech therapy is uncertain and
              slow, yet the patient is unlikely to live for more than a
              few months. The quickest and best palliation is
              Teflon® paste injection to the paralysed cord, which
              improves amplitude, prevents aspiration and enhances
              expectoration.
   e. True   Lymphatic spread is usually to the hilar nodes, but can
              occur in the supraclavicular nodes.

46. *Synopsis 517–518; Scott-Brown 5/8/9–10, 6/22/5–6*
   a. False   Tracheomalacia is a different condition. It exists in
              localized and generalized forms.
   b. False   The upper limit is 4–5 cm. The mediastinal trachea has
              to be mobilized and a laryngeal drop performed.
   c. False   Minor degrees of stenosis, with dyspnoea on exertion
              only, can safely be treated by repeat dilatations. The
              recurrent laryngeal nerve is at significant risk of
              damage from excision surgery.
   d. True   Grillo (USA) and Barclay (UK) described such a
              procedure for long stenoses. The stenotic segment is
              resected, and additional length is gained for primary
              anastomosis by resiting the right main bronchus into
              the left main bronchus.
   e. False   This is an indication for urgent thyroidectomy.

The mouth, pharynx and oesophagus

1. **Development of the mouth:**
   a. The stomatodeum, or primitive mouth, lies between frontonasal process cranially and first branchial arch caudally.
   b. The stomatodeum is lined by ectoderm.
   c. Cleft lip results from failure of fusion of the medial nasal, lateral nasal and maxillary processes.
   d. Failure of fusion of the palatal shelves of the maxillary processes results in cleft palate posterior to the incisive foramen.
   e. Rathke's pouch is an endodermal derivative which forms the posterior part of the pituitary gland.

2. **Development of the tongue:**
   a. The anterior two-thirds develops from the second branchial arch.
   b. The posterior one-third develops from the copula.
   c. Internal musculature is derived from suboccipital myotomes.
   d. The foramen caecum is the lingual opening of the thyroglossal duct.
   e. The glossopharyngeal nerve supplies third arch structures.

3. **Development of the pharynx:**
   a. The pharyngeal arches develop after the branchial arches.
   b. The glossopharyngeal nerve supplies second pouch derivatives.
   c. Tonsillar lymphatic tissue is of mesodermal origin.
   d. The cervical sinus (of His) normally communicates with the lumen of the pharynx.
   e. The hypopharynx is derived from the fifth pharyngeal pouch.

1. *Synopsis 3, 287–288; Scott-Brown 1/8/1–3, 6/19/10–13*
   a. True.
   b. True.
   c. True   The failure of fusion may be unilateral or bilateral, and may also result in cleft of the primary palate, anterior to the incisive foramen.
   d. True   This is cleft of the secondary palate.
   e. False   This is an cctodermal derivative that forms the anterior pituitary.

2. *Synopsis 3, 287; Scott-Brown 1/8/2–3*
   a. False   The anterior two-thirds is formed from the fusion of two lateral tubercles and the tuberculum impar. All are first arch derivatives.
   b. True   This is a midline derivative of the third arch, also known as the hypobranchial eminence.
   c. True   It is supplied by the hypoglossal nerve.
   d. True.
   e. True.

3. *Synopsis 3, 287–288; Scott-Brown 1/10/1–7*
   a. False   The terms are synonymous. Branchia are gills; humans do not develop gills, so the term pharyngeal arch is preferable.
   b. Truc   The facial nerve is also involved.
   c. True   All lymphatic tissue is of mesodermal origin.
   d. False   The cervical sinus is formed by a ventral overgrowth of the second arch, which comes to overlie the remaining arches and clefts caudal to it. It fuses with the neck skin (C2), burying the ectoderm of the third, fourth and sixth arches. There is normally no communication through the endodermal lining with the lumen of the pharynx. However, in some cases of branchial fistula, the endoderm does break down. It is usually the second pouch that does so, and therefore the internal opening of the fistula is above the tonsil.
   e. False   The fifth pouch disappears early, though it may form the ultimobranchial body, which may form the calcitonin-secreting C cells of the thyroid.

⌣ 4. **The second pharyngeal pouch:**
   a. This is lined with ectoderm.
   b. It has dorsal and ventral diverticula.
   c. It forms the whole of the Eustachian tube.
   d. It contributes to the formation of the middle ear.
   e. It forms the supratonsillar fossa.

5. **Anatomy of the mouth:**
   a. The vestibule is that part of the oral cavity in front of the molar teeth.
   b. The posterior limit of the oral cavity is the posterior faucial pillar (palatopharyngeal fold).
   c. The mouth is lined with stratified squamous epithelium.
   d. The parotid duct of Stensen opens opposite the lower second molar tooth.
   e. Mandibular and maxillary divisions of the trigeminal nerve supply the mouth.

6. **Dental anatomy:**
   a. The deciduous teeth consist of two incisors, one canine and two molars in each half jaw.
   b. There are 32 permanent teeth.
   c. Teeth develop from ectoderm only.
   d. The teeth of the upper jaw are supplied via the anterior, middle and posterior superior alveolar nerves.
   e. The apex of the root of the lower third molar lies below the mylohyoid line.

4. *Synopsis 3, 287–288; Scott-Brown 1/10/1–5*
   a. False All the pharyngeal pouches are lined by endoderm.
   b. True.
   c. False The Eustachian tube is derived from the first pouch
          (tubotympanic recess), with a contribution from the
          otic capsule.
   d. True The dorsal diverticulum becomes part of the
          tubotympanic recess. It carries a pretrematic nerve,
          the tympanic branch of the glossopharyngeal, into the
          middle ear.
   e. True.

5. *Synopsis 288; Scott-Brown 1/8/3–4, 5/3/1,12*
   a. False The vestibule is the space between the teeth and gums
          and the lips and cheeks. It opens into the oral cavity
          between the teeth and behind the last molars.
   b. False The anterior faucial pillar marks the boundary
          between mouth and oropharynx.
   c. True.
   d. False It opens opposite the upper second molar tooth.
   e. True The greater and lesser palatine nerves are from the
          maxillary division, the lingual from the mandibular.

6. *Synopsis 171, 289; Scott-Brown 1/8/17–23, 5/3/9*
   a. True.
   b. True There are two incisors, one canine, two premolars and
          three molars in each half jaw.
   c. False The enamel is ectodermal, but the dentine and
          cementum are mesodermal.
   d. True.
   e. True The clinical significance of this is that an apical abscess
          may point in the neck.

7. **Anatomy of the nasopharynx:**
   a. The lower boundary of the nasopharynx is the anterior faucial pillar.
   b. The Eustachian tube opens at the level of the inferior turbinate.
   √c. Squamous epithelium lines the normal nasopharynx.
   d. Passavant's muscle is made up of fibres of the palatopharyngeus.
   e. The internal carotid artery is in close relation to the lateral nasopharyngeal recess (fossa of Rosenmüller).

8. **Anatomy of the oropharynx:**
   a. The upper border of the oropharynx is at the level of the soft palate.
   b. The posterior third of the tongue is part of the oropharynx.
   c. The posterior boundary of the vallecula is the epiglottis.
   d. The oropharynx is lined with squamous epithelium.
   e. The palatine tonsil lies between the palatopharyngeal fold anteriorly and the palatoglossal fold posteriorly.

9. **The pharyngeal constrictor muscles:**
   √ a. The pharyngobasilar fascia lies outside the constrictors.
   b. The superior constrictor forms part of the tonsillar fossa.
   c. The middle constrictor has attachments to the hyoid bone and stylohyoid ligament.
   d. Killian's dehiscence is the gap between the middle and inferior constrictors.
   e. The motor nerve supply is from the pharyngeal plexus via accessory and vagus nerves, with cell bodies in the nucleus ambiguus.

7. *Synopsis 293–294; Scott-Brown 1/10/8–9*
   a. False   The lower boundary of the nasopharynx is the soft
              palate. The anterior faucial pillar demarcates mouth
              from oropharynx.
   b. True.
   c. False   It is lined with pseudostratified ciliated columnar
              (respiratory) epithelium.
   d. True   The lateral fibres pass inside superior constrictor and
              join posteriorly to form the velopharyngeal sphincter.
   e. True   This was a hazard of Eustachian tube catheterization, a
              procedure seldom performed since the advent of
              ventilation tubes (grommets).

8. *Synopsis 293–295; Scott-Brown 1/10/9–10, 5/14/1*
   a. True   The oropharynx extends from the junction of hard and
      ✓   soft palate to the floor of the vallecula at the level of the
              hyoid bone. It is bounded anteriorly by the palatoglossal
              fold, which demarcates it from the mouth. Until recently,
              UICC classification included the anterior wall of the
              epiglottis as part of the oropharynx. Tumours arising in this
              area are now regarded as supraglottic laryngeal tumours.
   b. True.
   c. True.
   d. True   It is lined with non-keratinizing stratified squamous
              epithelium.
   e. False   The palatopharyngeal fold is posterior and the
              palatoglossal anterior.

9. *Synopsis 296–298; Scott-Brown 1/10/18–20, 27, 5/10/2–3*
   a. False   It lies inside the constrictors.
   b. True   The fibres are seen during tonsillectomy, running obliquely
              across the fossa. They can be divided to gain access to
              the glossopharyngeal nerve in cases of glossopharyngeal
              neuralgia. An elongated styloid process is approached in
              the same way in the treatment of Eagle's syndrome.
   c. True   It originates in the acute angle formed by the stylohyoid
              ligament and the greater cornu of the hyoid.
   d. False   Killian's dehiscence is the potential gap that occurs
              posteriorly between the two parts of the inferior
              constrictor, the thyropharyngeus and cricopharyngeus.
              It is a weak point, and is the usual site of origin of a
              pharyngeal pouch (Zenker's diverticulum).
   e. True.

10. **Anatomy of the palatine tonsil:**
    a. The crypts are lined by squamous epithelium.
    ✓ b. There are no afferent lymphatics.
    c. The tonsillar artery is a branch of the greater palatine.
    d. Pain sensation from the tonsil is carried in the glossopharyngeal nerve.
    e. The size of the tonsil can be assessed accurately by looking in the mouth while using a tongue depressor.

11. **The parapharyngeal space:**
    ✓✓ a. This has no anatomical floor, allowing communication from skull base to superior mediastinum.
    b. There is free communication with the retropharyngeal space.
    c. The deep lobe of the parotid projects into its lateral wall.
    d. The contents include the carotid sheath, the lower four cranial nerves, and deep cervical lymph nodes.
    e. At the level of C5 vertebra, the lateral wall is formed by the sternomastoid muscle.

10. *Synopsis 300–303; Scott-Brown 1/10/22–26, 5/4/2–3, 6/18/9–10*
  a. True Non-keratinizing stratified squamous epithelium
           covers the pharyngeal surface and extends into all the
           crypts. Desquamated cells form part of the crypt
           debris, and can be seen as white or yellow spots.
  b. True The tonsil acts as an initial antigen-processing station for
           swallowed material, some of which is trapped in the crypts.
           Efferent lymphatics drain to the jugulodigastric node.
  c. False The tonsillar artery is a branch of the facial artery.
           Minor branches of the greater palatine artery supply
           the upper pole. Further blood supply is obtained from
           small branches of the lingual and ascending pharyngeal
           arteries.
  d. True Therefore, pain may be referred to the ear.
  e. False Some tonsils appear large because the tonsillar fossae
           are shallow, while others of similar or greater mass
           may be almost completely buried. In addition,
           contraction of the pharyngeal musculature can bring
           the tonsils closer to the midline, so the apparent size is
           variable in the individual patient. Tonsils that appear
           large are best described as 'prominent'.

11. *Synopsis 299–300, 350–351; Scott-Brown 1/15/9–10, 5/2/11–13,
  5/16/16, 5/22/2–3*
  a. True Infections can therefore spread intracranially and into
           the mediastinum. Conversely, middle ear infection can
           spread, via involvement of the jugular foramen or
           petrous apex, into the neck.
  b. False There is a condensation of fascia around the carotid
           sheath, which separates the parapharyngeal and
           retropharyngeal spaces. Bilateral spread of infection in
           the neck is rare.
  c. True A deep lobe parotid tumour is a common cause of a
           mass in the parapharyngeal space. These are usually
           situated anterior to the styloid process, whereas vascular
           and neurogenous tumours occur posteriorly – a helpful
           point in differential diagnosis by CT or MR scanning.
  d. True Other contents are the ascending pharyngeal and
           palatine arteries, the sympathetic chain and the styloid
           group of muscles.
  e. True In drainage of a parapharyngeal abscess, the approach
           is anterior to the sternomastoid for an abscess low in
           the neck, and posterior to the muscle for an abscess
           high in the neck.

12. **The retropharyngeal space:**
    a. This is bounded posteriorly by the prevertebral fascia, anteriorly by the buccopharyngeal fascia, and laterally by the carotid sheath.
    b. It extends from the skull base to the superior mediastinum.
    c. It contains the vertebral arteries.
    d. It contains the cervical nerve roots.
    e. A retropharyngeal abscess usually points in the anterior triangle of the neck.

13. **The glossopharyngeal nerve:**
    a. Roots emerge from the midbrain.
    b. It exits the skull via the anterior compartment of the jugular foramen.
    c. It supplies taste and common sensation to the posterior two-thirds of the tongue.
    d. Parasympathetic cell bodies for supply of the submandibular gland lie in the superior (petrous) ganglion.
    e. The tympanic branch (Jacobson's nerve) contains both sensory and parasympathetic secretomotor fibres.

14. **Lymphatic drainage of the pharynx:**
    a. All areas of the pharynx drain ultimately to the lower deep cervical group of nodes.
    b. The nasopharynx drains via retropharyngeal and upper deep cervical nodes.
    c. The tonsil drains to the jugulodigastric node.
    d. The base of the tongue has very little lymphatic drainage.
    e. The pyriform fossa may drain to paratracheal nodes.

12. *Synopsis 299–300, 351–353; Scott-Brown 1/10/25–26, 1/15/4, 5/4/5–6, 5/16/16, 6/18/3–4*
  a. True.
  b. True.
  c. False The space contains only loose alveolar tissue and the retropharyngeal lymph nodes of Rouvier.
  d. False.
  e. False The abscess may point into the pharynx, as a swelling on the posterior pharyngeal wall, or into the posterior triangle of the neck. An acute abscess is commoner in infants, and results from suppuration in the retropharyngeal lymph nodes following an upper respiratory tract infection. It is best drained through the mouth. A chronic abscess occurs in adults due to tuberculosis. The cervical vertebrae may be involved. If drainage is required, an external approach through the neck is necessary.

13. *Synopsis 533–534, 574, 586; Scott-Brown 1/16/21–22, 5/9/1,5–6*
  a. False Roots emerge from the hindbrain, between the olive and inferior cerebellar peduncle.
  b. True A fibrous septum of dura separates the glossopharyngeal nerve and inferior petrosal sinus from the vagus and accessory nerves. However, in clinical practice, a jugular foramen lesion will usually affect all three nerves.
  c. False It supplies the posterior one-third of the tongue, together with the tonsils, soft palate and middle ear. These are third arch and second pouch structures.
  d. False Parasympathetic cell bodies of the glossopharyngeal nerve are in the otic ganglion, and they supply the parotid. The submandibular gland is supplied from the nervus intermedius via the chorda tympani. The cell bodies in the petrous ganglion of the glossopharyngeal are sensory.
  e. True.

14. *Synopsis 304; Scott-Brown 1/10/22, 5/13/3, 5/15/3–4, 5/17/2–4*
  a. True.
  b. True.
  c. True.
  d. False There is rich bilateral drainage, hence the high incidence of neck metastases in carcinoma of the tongue base.
  e. True.

15. **Immunology of the pharyngeal lymphoid tissue:**
    a. B-lymphocytes proliferate in active follicles.
    b. T-lymphocytes secrete cytokines, which act locally to control the inflammatory response.
    c. B-lymphocytes synthesize IgA-secretory antibodies.
    d. Macrophages are involved in presenting antigen to T-lymphocytes.
    e. T4-lymphocytes required for cell-mediated immunity are found in excessive numbers in AIDS patients.

✓ 16. **The parotid gland:**
    a. Is covered on its outer aspect by a thickened layer of deep cervical fascia.
    b. The stylomandibular ligament forms a thick fascial barrier between the deep lobe and the parapharyngeal space.
    c. Secretomotor fibres to the gland travelling in the auriculotemporal nerve are involved in Frey's syndrome.
    ✓ d. The facial nerve trunk lies deep to the retromandibular vein.
    e. Developmental abnormalities of the ear are associated with a double trunk of the facial nerve in the parotid.

The mouth, pharynx and oesophagus

15. *Synopsis 312–313; Scott-Brown 1/18/6–16, 1/19/23–24*
    a. True   The follicles are similar to those found in lymph nodes,
            but in the pharyngeal lymphoid tissue there are no
            afferent lymphatics.
    b. True   Cytokines include migration inhibition factors (which
            localize macrophages and monocytes at the
            inflammatory site), macrophage activating factors, the
            interleukin series and the interferons.
    c. True   Some of these B-cells transform into plasma cells. The
            secretory IgA is joined into a dimeric form with a
            secretory protein by epithelial cells and is then
            released onto the lumenal surface of the mucosa.
            There it has neutralizing activity against viruses and
            toxins, and is able to inhibit many micro-organisms
            from adhering to the epithelial surface.
    d. True.
    e. False   T4-cell destruction due to HIV infection explains much
            of the pathology of AIDS. The T-cell is central in control
            of the entire immune response, but is particularly critical
            in dealing with micro-organisms that are able to 'take up
            residence' inside the cell. These include viruses,
            mycobacteria and protozoa. Cell-mediated immunity is
            also required to eliminate fungal infections.

16. *Synopsis 292–293, 373, 531; Scott-Brown 1/9/1–5, 1/15/9,
    5/2/18–20, 5/20/2–5*
    a. True   The thick, unyielding parotid fascia accounts for the severe
            pain of parotitis. It may also prevent a parotid swelling
            from becoming obvious until it has reached a large size.
    b. False   The stylomandibular ligament runs within the gland,
            separating the deep lobe from the superficial lobe anteriorly.
            It accounts for the 'dumb-bell' shape of tumours occupying
            both deep and superficial lobes. There is no significant
            fascial barrier between the deep lobe and the
            parapharyngeal space; hence, deep lobe tumours typically
            present as a parapharyngeal mass. The stylomandibular
            ligament is divided for access to a deep lobe tumour.
    c. True   Following parotidectomy these fibres may re-innervate
            sweat glands in the skin, leading to Frey's syndrome of
            gustatory sweating.
  ✓ d. False   The nerve is superficial to the vein. The external
            carotid artery is deeper still.
    e. True   Any developmental abnormality of the ear should alert
            the surgeon to the possibility of associated facial nerve
            anomalies.

17. The submandibular gland:
   a. The lingual nerve is attached to the superficial lobe by a fibrous band.
   b. The hyoglossus muscle divides deep from the superficial lobe.
   c. The duct runs between mylohyoid and hyoglossus to open laterally in the floor of the mouth opposite the second molar tooth.
   d. The mandibular division of the facial nerve lies superficial to the capsule of the gland.
   e. The facial artery can usually be retracted and kept intact during excision of the gland.

18. The infratemporal fossa:
   a. This lies below the posterior cranial fossa.
   b. It has no anatomical floor.
   c. The posterior boundary is the styloid apparatus and carotid sheath.
  √ d. The maxillary artery and maxillary nerve pass through the infratemporal fossa.
  √ e. It contains the pterygoid venous plexus.

19. The temporomandibular joint:
  √ a. This is a synovial joint.
   b. It allows both gliding and hinge movements.
  √ c. The medial pterygoid muscle inserts into the articular disc.
   d. Jaw opening is initiated by contraction of the lateral pterygoid muscle.
   e. Nerve supply is from the maxillary division of the trigeminal.

17. *Synopsis 293, 304, 373–374; Scott-Brown 1/9/4–6, 5/20/5*
    a. False   It is attached to the deep lobe by nerve fibres via the submandibular ganglion. The flat lingual nerve is pulled into a readily identifiable angular shape by downward retraction on the gland during dissection.
    b. False   The gland curls around the posterior border of the mylohyoid muscle. The mylohyoid defines the border between its lobes and is retracted forward during surgical excision. The hyoglossus lies deep to the gland in the floor of the mouth.
    c. False   The duct does run forward from the anterior aspect of the deep lobe, between the hyoglossus and mylohyoid, but opens near the midline at the base of the frenulum.
    d. True   This nerve, which supplies the corner of the mouth, is at risk during excision of the gland. It can be avoided by placing the incision just above the level of the hyoid and carrying out the dissection in the plane between gland and capsule.
    e. False   The facial artery normally has to be divided and ligated in two places. It runs forward and upward over the superficial lobe.

18. *Synopsis – no reference; Scott-Brown 1/5/28, 1/15/6–9, 5/2/9–11, 5/22/1–2, 8–9*
    a. False   It lies below the middle cranial fossa.
    b. True   It continues down into the neck and superior mediastinum.
    c. True.
    d. False   The maxillary artery and mandibular nerve pass through it.
    e. True   The plexus is formed around and within the lateral pterygoid muscle.

19. *Synopsis 290–291; Scott-Brown 1/8/9–11, 3/13/4, 4/22/10, 6/19/6–7*
    a. True.
    b. True   Hinge movements occur mainly in the lower compartment, sliding in the upper.
    c. False   The lateral pterygoid inserts into the articular disc.
    d. True   This muscle is inserted into a pit on the anterior border of the mandibular ramus just below the joint, and also into the articular disc.
    e. False   Supply is from the mandibular division, mainly from the auriculotemporal branch.

20. **The soft palate:**
    a. The palatine aponeurosis is formed by the expanded tendons of levator palati muscles.
    b. The tensor palati turns through 90° around the pterygoid hamulus.
    c. The soft palate contains mucous glands, lymphoid tissue and taste buds.
    d. It is lined by squamous epithelium on its superior surface.
    e. Its main blood supply comes from the greater palatine artery.

21. **Submucous cleft palate:**
    a. Velopharyngeal incompetence is easily diagnosed by intra-oral examination.
    b. A bifid uvula is pathognomonic of submucous cleft.
    c. A central posterior notch in the hard palate is a sign of submucous cleft.
    d. A submucous cleft is best treated by adenoidectomy.
    e. Associated glue ear is an absolute indication for adenoidectomy.

22. **White lesions of the oral cavity:**
    a. Leucoplakia can be rubbed off.
    b. Candidiasis may appear as a red or white area.
    c. Vitamin B_{12} deficiency causes white patches on the tongue.
    d. A pattern of red areas with white or yellow elevated borders that changes from day to day should be biopsied.
    e. A lace-like pattern is characteristic of lichen planus.

20. *Synopsis 170, 297; Scott-Brown 1/8/11–12, 1/10/11–17, 6/19/10, 18–26*
   a. False   It is formed by the expanded tendons of the tensor palati muscles, which meet in a midline raphe. This is the functional basis of the soft palate. All other muscles except the musculus uvulae insert into it.
   b. True.
   c. True.
   d. False   The upper (nasopharyngeal) surface is lined by respiratory epithelium, the lower by non-keratinizing stratified squamous epithelium.
   e. False   The main blood supply is from palatine branch of the ascending pharyngeal. The greater palatine artery supplies primarily the hard palate; it runs forward from the greater palatine foramen to the incisive canal.

21. *Synopsis 200, 296, 322; Scott-Brown 6/19/13–30*
   a. False   Diagnosis is difficult by this method unless there is a gross degree of incompetence. It is best diagnosed by rigid nasal endoscopy using an angled lens.
   b. False   Although most cases of submucous cleft also have a bifid uvula, isolated bifid uvula is common (1 per cent of population). Most cases of bifid uvula are not associated with submucous cleft.
   c. True   This is a more reliable sign than bifid uvula.
   d. False   An asymptomatic or occult submucous cleft may be rendered overt following adenoidectomy, as the mass of adenoids was helping maintain velopharyngeal competence. A submucous cleft is a contraindication to adenoidectomy.
   e. False   See above.

22. *Synopsis 328–331; Scott-Brown 5/3/2–8*
   a. False   The definition of leucoplakia is a white patch which cannot be rubbed off.
   b. True.
   c. False   This causes a red, beefy tongue.
   d. False   The description is of geographical tongue, and management consists of reassurance.
   e. True   This is not always present; the oral lesions may be simple white plaques. There may also be pinkish patches on the skin.

23. **Mouth ulcers:**
    a. Giant aphthous ulcers occur in AIDS.
    b. Herpes simplex ulceration in children may be complicated by acute encephalitis.
    √ c. Ulcers of the mouth and genitalia with uveitis characterize Reiter's syndrome.
    d. Local steroids are used in the treatment of aphthous ulcers.
    √ e. Pemphigus vulgaris should be treated by masterly inactivity.

24. **Tumours of the mouth:**
    a. An epulis is a midline bony lesion of the hard palate.
    b. Papilloma is caused by a DNA virus.
    c. Minor salivary gland tumours are almost always benign.
    d. A chronic ulcer in the floor of the mouth is likely to be malignant.
    e. Carcinoma is commoner on the lower lip than the upper.

25. **Salivary gland tumours:**
    a. The commonest parotid tumour is the adenoid cystic carcinoma.
    b. The adenolymphoma (Warthin's tumour) is commoner in young women, is painful and grows rapidly.
    c. A submandibular tumour is more likely to be malignant than a parotid tumour.
    d. In muco-epidermoid carcinoma, recurrence rates and survival correlate with histological grade.
    e. Distant metastases after many years are characteristic of adenoid cystic carcinoma.

The mouth, pharynx and oesophagus

23. *Synopsis 323–331; Scott-Brown 5/3/2–6*
 a. True   Pain is the major symptom, and can be severe.
 b. True   Intravenous aciclovir is used to treat this complication.
 c. False   The description is of Behçet's syndrome. Reiter's is characterized by iritis and arthritis following either urethritis or dysentery.
 d. True   They are administered either as pellets, to be sucked, or as a paste applied directly.
 e. False   If treated with masterly inactivity, it is likely to be followed by forced inactivity, as the condition is fatal without aggressive steroid treatment!

24. *Synopsis 358–362; Scott-Brown 5/3/8–28*
 a. False   An epulis is any soft tissue swelling of the gums. The midline bony swelling of the palate is the torus palatinus.
 b. True   It is caused by the human papilloma virus. There are various strains, each with a penchant for certain sites.
 c. False   50 per cent are malignant, mainly adenoid cystic carcinoma.
 d. True   This is the so-called 'sump area'.
 e. True   This is probably because of exposure to sunlight, and it is commoner in outdoor workers.

25. *Synopsis 373–374; Scott-Brown 5/20/6–9, 5/21/2–8, 6/32/11–13*
 a. False   The commonest type is pleomorphic adenoma (mixed parotid tumour), which accounts for 80 per cent of cases.
 b. False   85 per cent of these tumours occur in males, mostly aged 50–70 years. They are slow growing and painless, and are bilateral in 10 per cent of cases. They characteristically occur in the tail of the parotid and are soft, sometimes fluctuant.
 c. True   20 per cent of parotid tumours and 40 per cent of submandibular tumours are malignant. However, because parotid tumours are much commoner than submandibular (ratio 10:1), the overall incidence of malignant parotid tumours is greater than that of malignant submandibular tumours.
 d. True   Low-grade muco-epidermoid carcinoma recurs locally in 6 per cent of cases and has a 90 per cent 5-year survival rate, whereas the high-grade type recurs in up to 80 per cent of patients and only 20 per cent survive 5 years. In addition, metastasis is rare in low-grade tumours but occurs in 60 per cent of high-grade tumours.
 e. True   These are commonest in the lung, and may recur up to 20 years after apparently successful removal of the primary.

√ 26. **Benign salivary gland disease:**
    a. Calculi occur more commonly in the mucus-secreting salivary glands than in the serous.
    b. Unilateral parotid gland enlargement may occur in mumps.
    c. Mikulicz syndrome consists of bilateral enlargement of the lacrimal, parotid and submandibular glands.
    d. Sjögren's syndrome has the same salivary gland changes as Mikulicz syndrome in association with a connective tissue disease, usually rheumatoid arthritis.
    e. Malignant lymphoma arising in the affected salivary glands is a recognized complication of Sjögren's syndrome.

27. **During deglutition:**
    a. Elevation of the hyoid bone reduces the size of the oval cavity.
    b. Passavant's bar assists closure of the nasopharyngeal hiatus.
√ c. A fixed thyroid cartilage is necessary in the pharyngeal phase.
    d. The epiglottis directs the food stream into two lateral channels.
    e. A peristaltic wave starts in the top of the pharynx as the bolus enters the oesophagus.

26. *Synopsis 314; Scott-Brown 5/19/3–11, 6/32/6–9*
   a. True   Approximately 80 per cent occur in the submandibular
            gland, which is mainly mucus-secreting. Stones are rare
            in the parotid, which is mainly serous.
   b. True   Enlargement is usually bilateral, but can be unilateral.
            Orchitis, pancreatitis and hepatitis may be associated.
   c. True   This was first described by Mikulicz in 1888. The term
            'benign lymphoepithelial lesion' was proposed by
            Godwin in 1952, and is now preferred.
   d. True   This was described by Henrik Sjögren, a Stockholm
   √   ophthalmologist, in 1933. Keratoconjunctivitis sicca
            and xerostomia with enlargement of salivary and
            lacrimal glands are the main symptoms. It occurs in
            association with rheumatoid arthritis, polymyositis,
            systemic lupus erythematosus, scleroderma and
            polyarteritis nodosa.
   e. True   This is more likely to occur in those cases presenting
            with salivary gland enlargement.

27. *Synopsis 315–316; Scott-Brown 1/11/3–7*
   a. True   This ensures that elevation of the tongue from before
            backwards forces the food bolus posteriorly into the
            pharynx.
   b. True   Contraction of the laterally placed palatopharyngeal
            muscles produces this ridge and assists closure by
            approximating with the elevated soft palate (levator
            and tensor palatini).
   c. False Closure of the laryngeal inlet is effected by elevation of
            the larynx under the shelter of the tongue base. A fixed
            cartilage would allow aspiration of food. Other factors
            in closure of the laryngeal isthmus include inhibition of
            respiration, closure of laryngeal sphincters
            (aryepiglottic folds, thyro-arytenoid muscles and false
            cords), and the action of the epiglottis.
   d. True   Food is directed toward the pyriform fossae.
   e. True   This wave travels caudally and clears food behind the
            bolus and also produces contraction of the
            cricopharyngeus to prevent regurgitation.

28. **Pathophysiology of swallowing:**
    a. In bulbar palsy, swallowing of liquids is characteristically more difficult than swallowing solids.
    b. A vagal paralysis has its main clinical effect on the oesophageal phase of swallowing.
    c. Cricopharyngeal myotomy is of no benefit if the cause of dysphagia is neurological.
    d. Globus pharyngis may be associated with gastro-oesophageal reflux.
    e. The main disadvantage of milk nasendoscopy compared with videofluoroscopy is that it cannot reliably detect aspiration.

29. **Stertor:**
    a. Stertor is defined as noisy respiration due to partial airway obstruction below the level of the epiglottis.
    b. The Venturi effect is implicated in causing the noise.
    c. The noise is loudest on expiration.
    d. Intercostal recession is a feature of severe stertor.
    e. Large tonsils and adenoids may be causative of stertor.

28. *Synopsis 386, 397, 485–486,574–577; Scott-Brown 1/12/10–15, 5/9/1–10, 5/24/2–3,24–25*

   a. True   In particular, aspiration is more of a problem.

   b. False The major clinical effect is seen in the pharyngeal phase, especially failure of laryngeal closure leading to aspiration.

   c. False The operation is of benefit in cases where failure of relaxation or spasm are causing symptoms; many of these will be neurological in origin.

   d. True   However, no definite causal link has been proven. Antacid medication is effective in some cases.

   e. False Both methods will reliably detect aspiration. Milk nasendoscopy cannot demonstrate the oral and oesophageal phases of swallowing, which are seen well on videofluoroscopy. It is, however, cheaper and quicker, and can be repeated without radiation exposure.

29. *Synopsis 387; Scott-Brown 6/21/1–9*

   a. False It is due to partial airway obstruction above the level of the larynx.

   b. True   The Venturi effect is the fall in lateral pressure exerted by a gas when it moves along a tube. The fall in pressure is greater if the flow per unit area is increased because of narrowing of the tube. If the walls of the tube are not sufficiently rigid they will collapse inward; the flow then ceases and the pressure drop returns to normal. This cycle, rapidly repeated, causes the noise of stertor.

   c. False Stertor occurs on inspiration. On expiration, the intramural pressure is greater than extramural.

   d. True.

   e. True   Large tonsils and adenoids are probably the commonest cause of stertor.

30. **Obstructive sleep apnoea syndrome:**
    a. This is defined as the cessation of airflow at the nose and mouth with cessation of respiratory effort.
    b. It is associated with failure to thrive and feeding difficulties in the infant.
    c. Bradycardia is a sign of minor importance.
    d. The Müller manoeuvre is performed with the flexible fibreoptic laryngoscope during induction of anaesthesia.
    e. In Pierre-Robin syndrome, the respiratory obstruction is most likely to occur in the prone position.

31. **Diphtheria:**
    a. This is caused by *Mycobacterium diphtheriae*, which is a normal commensal of the upper airways in 30 per cent of the UK population.
    b. Vaccination is ineffective.
    c. An endotoxin is responsible for death by myocarditis.
    d. The membrane is easily removed by swabbing.
    e. In suspected cases, treatment is deferred pending the results of a Schick test.

The mouth, pharynx and oesophagus

30. *Synopsis 387–389; Scott-Brown 5/4/15–16, 6/20/1–10*
    a. False One definition of sleep apnoea is the occurrence of 30
       or more episodes of apnoea, each being a cessation of
       airflow for more than 10 s, over a 7-hour sleep period.
       In obstructive sleep apnoea, respiratory efforts persist
       and are recordable as chest wall movements. In central
       sleep apnoea there is no respiratory effort.
    b. True.
    c. False Bradycardia implies a dangerous degree of hypoxaemia
       requiring urgent measures to restore an adequate airway.
    d. False The Müller manoevre is a 'reverse Valsalva',
       performed by the conscious patient while the examiner
       looks for the level of obstruction with the flexible
       fibreoptic laryngoscope. Sleep nasendoscopy is
       performed during induction of anaesthesia.
    e. False Pierre-Robin syndrome is cleft palate and micrognathia.
       Respiratory obstruction is most likely in the supine
       position. The position of choice for nursing the
       affected neonate is prone.

31. *Synopsis 336, 457; Scott-Brown 1/19/7–8, 4/8/25,33–4, 5/4/6–7,
    5/9/6–7, 6/24/5–6*
    a. False Diphtheria is caused by *Corynebacterium diphtheriae*, of
       which there are several strains, mitis being least serious
       and gravis the most serious. These are not the same as
       the 'diphtheroid' organisms, which are common
       commensals in the upper air and food passages.
    b. False The vaccine is given as part of the 'triple vaccine' (diphtheria/
       pertussis/tetanus) to infants at 3, 6 and 9 months of age.
       It has been a very successful public health measure.
       Diphtheria is now a rare disease in the UK, but cases do
       occur in unvaccinated patients and immigrants.
    c. False An exotoxin is responsible for death by myocarditis.
    d. False The membrane is characteristically thick, grey and
       adherent. Removal causes bleeding.
    e. False If the condition is suspected, antitoxin must be given
       urgently because of the risk of sudden death from
       myocarditis or respiratory obstruction. The Schick test
       is a test to determine susceptibility. A purified
       derivative of toxin is injected into the skin and the
       local inflammatory response noted. The test has a role
       in screening contacts after an outbreak to determine
       whether immunization is required.

32. **Chronic non-specific pharyngitis:**
    a. This is associated with smoking.
    b. It is exacerbated by chronic bronchitis.
    c. Lymphoid hypertrophy is seen in some cases.
    d. Tonsillectomy is the treatment of choice.
    e. The patient should be encouraged to clear the throat regularly to prevent a build-up of irritating thick catarrh.

33. **Chronic specific pharyngitis:**
    a. A gumma is a feature of secondary syphilis.
    b. Serological tests for syphilis are often negative in the presence of a chancre.
    c. Tuberculosis may cause painful pharyngeal ulceration.
    d. Scarring does not occur if tuberculosis is treated with antituberculous drugs.
    e. Lepromatous ulcers are usually painless.

34. **Acute tonsillitis:**
    a. Peak incidence is in the 1–3 years age group.
    b. A preceding viral infection of the upper respiratory tract is a predisposing factor.
    c. The alpha-haemolytic streptococcus is the commonest bacterial cause.
    d. Enlargement of the jugulodigastric lymph nodes is rarely seen except in glandular fever.
    e. In infectious mononucleosis (glandular fever), the absolute lymphocyte count is reduced.

32. *Synopsis 338; Scott-Brown 5/4/10–11, 5/24/25–27*
   a. True.
   b. True   This is due to the repeated physical trauma of coughing and the chronic presence of infected sputum.
   c. True   The pharyngeal wall appears granular, often with prominent lateral pharyngeal bands.
   d. False   Tonsillectomy is of no benefit unless the tonsils themselves are inflamed. Chronic pharyngitis is common in patients who have already had tonsillectomy.
   e. False   Throat-clearing is detrimental. It exacerbates and perpetuates the condition, and should be discouraged.

33. *Synopsis 340–343; Scott-Brown 5/4/11–13*
   a. False   A gumma is seen in tertiary syphilis. Snail-track ulcers (symmetrically placed), mucous patches and rubbery cervical lymphadenopathy are the characteristic features of secondary syphilis.
   b. True   The diagnosis is made by examining a smear taken from the lesion under dark ground illumination, when the spirochaetes will be seen.
   c. True.
   d. False   Severe scarring with stenosis occurs despite treatment.
   e. True   This is because the peripheral nerve endings are destroyed.

34. *Synopsis 345–347; Scott-Brown 5/4/2–3, 6/18/1–2*
   a. False   Peak incidence is between 4 and 6 years of age.
   b. True.
   c. False   Beta-haemolytic streptococcus is the commonest bacterial cause.
   d. False   Enlargement of the local nodes is very common.
   e. False   There is a lymphocytosis, with the presence of atypical lymphocytes. The Paul-Bunnell test is positive.

35. Quinsy:
  a. This is defined as a peritonsillar abscess.
  b. It is commonest in children.
  c. The pus lies in the space between the superior constrictor muscle and the carotid sheath.
  d. Trismus and dribbling are clinical features.
  e. Treatment consists of systemic antibiotics and drainage.

36. Tonsillectomy:
  a. Indications include central sleep apnoea.
  b. A family history of bleeding is an absolute contraindication.
  c. The dissection method is quicker than the guillotine.
  d. The Boyle-Davis gag with Doughty modification is used with nasotracheal intubation.
  e. A major arterial bleed can occur from the facial artery.

37. Benign tumours of the oropharynx:
  a. The commonest benign tumour of the oropharynx is the squamous cell papilloma.
  b. A virus is implicated in the aetiology of squamous cell papilloma.
  c. A smooth swelling of the lateral wall should be biopsied transorally.
  d. Most tonsillar tumours are benign.
  e. Salivary gland tumours rarely occur in the soft palate.

35. *Synopsis 349–350; Scott-Brown 5/4/3–4, 6/18/2*
  a. True.
  b. False Quinsy is commonest in young adults.
  c. False This would be a parapharyngeal abscess, which may complicate a quinsy. In a quinsy, the pus lies in the space between the tonsil capsule and the pharyngeal wall (superior constrictor muscle).
  d. True.
  e. True Drainage may be carried out by incision under surface anaesthesia. Quinsy tonsillectomy is an alternative, but is rarely performed.

36. *Synopsis 309, 354–358; Scott-Brown 5/4/17–23, 6/18/7–12*
  a. False Indications include obstructive sleep apnoea.
  b. False A family history of bleeding is an indication for studies of clotting profile.
  c. False The guillotine method is quicker; however, dissection is more precise, more thorough and has fewer complications, and is therefore preferred.
  d. False The Doughty modification is the split blade for the gag, and is for the orotracheal tube. Adenoidectomy, which is often combined with tonsillectomy in children, cannot be done with a nasotracheal tube.
  e. True The facial artery loops just lateral to the superior constrictor and can be damaged during dissection of a fibrotic tonsillar bed, particularly in adults.

37. *Synopsis 366; Scott-Brown 5/14/1–3*
  a. True.
  b. True The human papilloma virus is implicated.
  c. False The swelling may be a deep lobe parotid tumour, a neurogenous tumour, a paraganglioma or a carotid aneurysm. These will require an external approach following pre-operative CT or MRI evaluation.
  d. False Most are malignant, either squamous carcinoma or lymphoma.
  e. True They are commoner on the hard palate, which is part of the oral cavity.

38. Malignant tumours of the oropharynx:
  a. Sites include the faucial pillars, soft palate, tonsil, base of tongue, vallecula and posterior pharyngeal wall.
  b. The commonest site is the base of the tongue.
  c. Squamous carcinoma, lymphoma and salivary gland tumours occur in that order of frequency.
  d. Lymph node metastases are rare in squamous carcinoma.
  e. The jugulodigastric lymph nodes are the commonest site for metastases.

39. Lymphoma of the oropharynx:
  a. Most cases are Hodgkin's.
  b. The B-cell is the commonest cell of origin.
  c. Burkitt's lymphoma is associated with the herpes simplex virus.
  d. Investigations should include exploratory laparotomy.
  e. Complete surgical excision is the treatment of choice.

38. *Synopsis 367–368; Scott-Brown 5/14/1–18*
  a. True   The anterior (lingual) surface of the epiglottis was included in the UICC classification. The AJC system always regarded this as part of the larynx (suprahyoid epiglottis). It is now agreed as being part of the larynx.
  b. False   The commonest site is the tonsil (50 per cent). Base of tongue tumours account for around 25 per cent of cases.
  c. True   Frequency of occurrence is 70 per cent, 25 per cent and 5 per cent respectively.
  d. False   Nodal metastases occur in at least 60 per cent of cases.
  e. True   Around 75 per cent of metastases occur in the jugulodigastric lymph nodes.

39. *Synopsis 369; Scott-Brown 5/14/5–8,17–18*
  a. False   The majority are non-Hodgkin's and of high-grade malignancy.
  b. True.
  c. False   It is associated with the Epstein-Barr virus.
  d. False   This is not necessary with modern radiological techniques, e.g. abdominal CT scanning.
  e. False   Complete excision is unlikely to be achieved. These tumours are particularly sensitive to radiotherapy and chemotherapy, and combinations of the two are the treatment of choice.

40. **Treatment of squamous carcinoma of the tonsil:**
    a. Surgery is of no benefit if there are lymph node metastases.
    b. Radiotherapy is only given for palliation.
    c. The general condition of the patient is of major prognostic significance.
    d. A pectoralis major myocutaneous flap gives better speech and swallowing rehabilitation results than a radial forearm free flap with microvascular anastomosis.
    e. Cisplatin has effectively cured some advanced cases in Phase 3 trials, but at the cost of ototoxicity.

41. **Hypopharyngeal tumours:**
    a. Sites include the pyriform fossa, post-cricoid region and vallecula.
    b. Benign tumours are common.
    c. Post-cricoid carcinoma is commoner in women.
    d. Pyriform fossa tumours spread laterally into the paraglottic space.
    e. A T3 tumour is associated with a fixed vocal cord and means that the recurrent laryngeal nerve has been invaded.

40. *Synopsis 368; Scott-Brown 5/14/10–17*
   a. False   Radical neck dissection is the best available treatment for neck node metastases, provided they are unilateral, not fixed and less than 6 cm in diameter. It can be carried out in continuity with removal of the primary in a COMMANDO operation (COMbined neck dissection, MANDibulectomy and resection of Oropharynx).
   b. False   Cure can be achieved with radiotherapy alone in favourable cases, i.e. a small tumour with no nodes and the patient in generally good condition. Radiotherapy is also used in combination with surgical excision in planned combined treatment, which gives 5-year survival rates of the order of 30 per cent.
   c. True.
   d. False   The free flap gives better functional results, but the myocutaneous flap is technically easier and is therefore a more reliable procedure in less experienced hands.
   e. False   Survival times have been extended in some studies by a few months; unfortunately, this is well short of cure. Ototoxicity does occur, as well as more serious and life-threatening side effects due to suppression of the immune system.

41. *Synopsis 370–373; Scott-Brown 5/15/1–15*
   a. False   The hypopharynx extends from the level of the hyoid bone to the lower border of the cricoid cartilage. The vallecula is part of the oropharynx. The third hypopharyngeal site is the posterior pharyngeal wall, between the level of the floor of the vallecula and the cricoarytenoid joints.
   b. False   99 per cent of these tumours are malignant; nearly all are squamous carcinoma.
   c. True   The ratio of women to men is 2:1.
   d. False   The paraglottic space is medial to the pyriform fossa. Lateral spread is via the thyrohyoid membrane.
   e. False   Cord fixation is present in T3 tumours, but does not necessarily mean recurrent laryngeal nerve involvement. Fixation could be caused by invasion of muscles or of the cricoarytenoid joint.

42. **Carcinoma of the pyriform fossa:**
    a. This is commonest in males aged 50–70 years.
    b. Dysphagia with pain on swallowing radiating to the ear is characteristic.
    c. Presentation as a neck node with an unknown primary is not uncommon.
    d. Occult nodal metastases are present in over 30 per cent of clinically non-palpable necks.
    e. Surgical treatment usually allows preservation of the larynx.

43. **Total pharyngolaryngectomy:**
    a. The main indication for total pharyngolaryngectomy is squamous carcinoma of the post-cricoid region.
    b. Primary anastomosis of the orostome to the cervical oesophagus is achieved in the majority of cases.
    c. The thyroid gland is removed during the surgery.
    d. The pectoralis major myocutaneous flap can be used for reconstruction.
    e. The free jejunal graft with microvascular anastamosis is only suitable for disease confined to the neck.

44. **Total pharyngolaryngectomy and oesophagectomy:**
    a. Gastric transposition necessitates cervical, thoracic and abdominal incisions.
    b. Colon transposition has the disadvantage of three anastomoses.
    c. Stenosis is the main complication of using stomach for the repair.
    d. Post-operative thyroid and calcium supplements are required.
    e. A pneumothorax is treated by insertion of a chest drain.

42. *Synopsis 370–373; Scott-Brown 5/15/1–15*
 a. True.
 b. True.
 c. True.
 d. True.
 e. False Total laryngectomy is required because the larynx is nearly always invaded via the paraglottic space. Also, if there is an insufficient margin of uninvolved pharyngeal mucosa to allow primary closure of an adequate food passage, a total laryngopharyngectomy with pharyngeal reconstruction will be required.

43. *Synopsis 310–311, 371–373, 409; Scott-Brown 5/15/8–15*
 a. True It is also indicated for extensive pyriform fossa carcinoma lesions and upper oesophageal tumours.
 b. False This manoeuvre is not a practical surgical option because of the segmental blood supply of the oesophagus. In addition, there is frequently extensive submucosal spread of disease in the oesophagus, so oesophagectomy is desirable on oncological grounds.
 c. True.
 d. True.
 e. True.

44. *Synopsis 371–373; Scott-Brown 5/15/8–15*
 a. False Thoracic incision is not necessary; the thoracic oesophagus can be freed by blind finger dissection from below, and the mobilized stomach can be passed up in a similar way. However, there is a risk of massive haemorrhage, and the surgical team must be prepared to do an immediate thoracotomy if required.
 b. True One is in the neck, one is between the lower end of the transposed colon and the stomach, and one is to restore continuity between the ileum and the descending colon (the caecum and terminal ileum are discarded).
 c. False Stenosis is very rare. The main complication is the operative mortality (5–25 per cent).
 d. True This is because the thyroid and parathyroids are removed.
 e. True An underwater seal chest drain is used.

45. Recurrence of hypopharyngeal carcinoma:
    a. Distant metastases are the usual cause of death.
 ✓ b. Regular follow-up examination provides reliable early detection.
    c. Possible causes include tumour implantation at operation.
    d. Stomal recurrence can be treated by thoracotracheostomy with manubrial resection, but this is rarely successful.
    e. Recurrence may present as a persistent pharyngocutaneous fistula.

46. Malignant cervical lymph nodes:
    a. Assessment for TNM staging by palpation is subject to inter-observer variation of around 30 per cent among trained specialists.
    b. CT scanning can reliably distinguish nodes containing tumour from reactive nodes.
    c. Non-palpable nodes containing tumour (clinically occult metastases) may be detected on ultrasound-guided fine needle aspiration cytology.
    d. Nodes in the supraclavicular fossa carry a worse prognosis than nodes in the submandibular triangle.
    e. Because of the unreliability of clinical assessment, N-status is unrelated to prognosis.

47. Radical neck dissection:
    a. This consists of removal of all the lymph-bearing structures between the midline, mandible, anterior border of the sternomastoid and the clavicle.
    b. The sternomastoid muscle, internal jugular vein and submandibular gland are excised with the specimen.
 ✓ c. The upper end of the internal jugular vein is divided first.
    d. In the standard radical operation, the accessory nerve is preserved.
    e. A chylous leak during a left-sided operation is recognized as milky fluid collecting in the lower part of the wound.

45. *Synopsis 370–373; Scott-Brown 5/15/1–15*
  a. False Loco-regional recurrence at the primary site, resection margins and cervical nodes is the commonest cause of death.
  b. False Early detection is difficult because of the radiotherapy reaction and scarring which follows earlier therapy.
  c. True.
  d. True.
  e. True.

46. *Synopsis 308, 435; Scott-Brown 5/2/13, 5/15/6–10, 5/17/5–7*
  a. True.
  b. False CT scanning can reliably detect enlarged nodes, but these do not necessarily contain tumour. CT signs such as central necrosis, capsule enhancement and poorly-defined margins do correlate with malignancy, but may also be found in the presence of infection. CT is useful in assessing patients with short, thick necks, which are difficult to palpate accurately.
  c. True Success is highly operator-dependent, but this is a useful tool in skilled hands. In oropharyngeal, hypopharyngeal and supraglottic laryngeal primaries (T2 and greater), there is a high risk of occult nodal metastases.
  d. True.
  e. False N-status correlates well with prognosis; there is little difficulty with classifying patients who have large, multiple, fixed or bilateral nodes, and these have a very poor prognosis.

47. *Synopsis 435; Scott-Brown 5/17/8–15*
  a. False Anterior border of trapezius, not sternomastoid. The area described is the anterior triangle only.
  b. True.
  c. False The lower end is divided first, to prevent tumour embolization during subsequent dissection.
  d. False The accessory nerve is divided at the anterior border of the trapezius. Many surgeons will, however, attempt to preserve it in an otherwise radical operation, provided there is no obvious malignancy in its vicinity.
  e. False The patient will have been starved, so the chyle is clear.

48. **Functional or conservation neck dissection:**
    a. This aims to remove only the nodes and tissue likely to be involved by tumour.
    b. Published indications include the clinically N0 neck with a high risk of occult metastases.
    c. Papillary carcinoma of the thyroid is a generally accepted indication.
    d. The accessory nerve is preserved.
    e. In the Bocca operation, the sternomastoid is preserved.

49. **Pharyngeal pouch (Zenker's diverticulum):**
    a. Its origin is between the middle and inferior constrictor muscles (dehiscence of Killian).
    b. The cause is traction by contracting tuberculous scar tissue.
    c. Associated symptoms include dysphagia and dyspnoea.
    ✓ d. Dohlman's operation is an endoscopic excision of the pouch.
    e. Inversion of the pouch is an alternative to excision.

50. **Thyroglossal cysts and sinuses:**
    a. These result from developmental abnormalities of the descent of the thyroid from the foramen caecum.
    b. They usually present as a midline neck swelling in a child or young adult.
    c. The majority of them are above the level of the hyoid.
    d. An infected cyst should be incised and drained.
    e. In Sistrunk's operation, the entire hyoid bone is removed.

48. *Synopsis 435; Scott-Brown 5/17/12–13*
a. True   The risk is that unrecognized tumour will be left behind.
b. True   The argument against elective neck dissection in general is that survival is not improved compared with a 'wait and see' policy, with surgery for recurrences.
c. True.
d. True   The accessory nerve is preserved, plus or minus the sternomastoid muscle, internal jugular vein, cervical plexus and submandibular gland.
e. True   This operation also preserves the internal jugular vein and accessory nerve.

49. *Synopsis 297, 380–382; Scott-Brown 5/10/1–19*
a. False   The dehiscence is between the two parts of the inferior constrictor: the thyropharyngeus and cricopharyngeus.
b. False   It is a pulsion diverticulum; raised intrapharyngeal pressure causes bulging of mucosa through the weak zone posteriorly. There is failure of normal coordination of swallowing, but the underlying cause of this is not known.
c. True   Dysphagia is an early symptom; dyspnoea comes later because of aspiration pneumonia.
d. False   This is endoscopic diathermy division of the party wall between diverticulum and oesophagus. Special instruments are required.
e. True   It is easier, there is less risk of infection (since the pharynx is not opened) or stricture, and less risk of damaging the recurrent laryngeal nerve. There is a small risk of developing a carcinoma on the inverted sac mucosa.

50. *Synopsis 287, 322; Scott-Brown 5/16/1–4, 6/30/8–12*
a. True.
b. True   90 per cent are midline; 66 per cent in patients under 30 years of age. The lump moves up on protruding the tongue and on swallowing.
c. False   Only 25 per cent are suprahyoid.
d. False   This makes subsequent excision difficult. It should be treated with antibiotics, with definitive excision as an elective procedure. Needle aspiration is a useful method for dealing with the acute episode, but if the contents are very viscid this may not be possible.
e. False   Only the body of the hyoid is removed.

51. Branchial sinuses and fistulae:
   a. The majority of these are present at birth.
   b. An internal opening in the supratonsillar fossa implies the origin is from the cervical sinus of His.
   c. A tract passing between the internal and external carotid arteries suggests the origin is from the first branchial cleft.
   d. A collaural fistula has two openings.
   e. First-line treatment consists of injection of sclerosants.

52. Branchial cysts:
   a. Most branchial cysts are associated with internal openings.
   b. Histology supports the theory of their origin from squamous cell rests within lymph nodes.
   c. The peak age of onset is 20–30 years.
   d. Aspiration should never be performed because of the risk of implanting cholesterol crystals in the neck.
   e. Hodgkin's disease is part of the differential diagnosis.

51. *Synopsis 375–376; Scott-Brown 5/16/4–7, 6/30/2–6*
a. True   Branchial cysts, however, usually present in early adult life.
b. False   This implies the origin is from the second pharyngeal pouch. The cervical sinus is formed by a ventral overgrowth of the second arch, which comes to overlie the remaining arches and clefts caudal to it. It fuses with the neck skin (C2), burying the ectoderm of the third, fourth and sixth arches. There is not normally any communication with the lumen of the pharynx.
c. False   It suggests the origin is from the second pouch. First branchial pouch abnormalities may account for cysts high in the neck and for fistulae opening in the external auditory meatus.
d. True   Any true fistula has two openings. The collaural fistula passes between the external auditory meatus and the skin of the neck, opening between the angle of the mandible and the sternomastoid. It is probably a first cleft defect.
e. False   Treatment, if required, is excision of the whole tract.

52. *Synopsis 375–6 ; Scott-Brown 5/16/4–7, 6/30/1–4*
a. False   This is a rare occurrence.
b. True   Most branchial cysts are lined with squamous epithelium and have lymphoid tissue in their walls.
c. True.
d. False   This is nonsense.
e. True   Other lymphomas, secondary deposits, paraganglioma, tuberculosis and reactive lymphadenitis must also be considered.

53. **The adult oesophagus:**
    a. The pharynx joins the oesophagus at the glosso-epiglottic folds.
    b. There are only two constrictions along its length.
    c. The non-striated muscle has a motor supply from the vagus.
    d. Portal-systemic anastomoses are located in the middle third.
    e. The cricopharyngeal sphincter is about 3 cm in length.

54. **The lower oesophageal sphincter:**
    a. This can be demonstrated histologically.
    b. A pinch-cock effect is produced by the left crus of the diaphragm.
    c. Mucosal folds at the lower end of the oesophagus may form a valve.
    d. A normal oesophagogastric angle prevents acid reflux.
    e. The sling of Willis is essential in sphincteric action.

53. *Synopsis 393–396; Scott-Brown 1/10/28–39, 5/24/1–2*

a. False The oesophagus starts and the pharynx ends at the lower border of the cricoid cartilage, which is at the level of C6 in adults.

b. False There are three constrictions, and each one may be a site of impaction of a foreign body. Starting from the incisor teeth they are: at 15 cm, the cricopharyngeal sphincter; at 25 cm, where the aortic arch and left main bronchus cross the oesophagus; and at 40 cm, the region of the gastro-oesophageal sphincter.

c. True This is true of the lower two-thirds of the oesophagus. It is mainly parasympathetic, and the cell bodies are in the vagal nucleus. The upper third is striated and is supplied by the recurrent nerves.

d. False They are located in the lower third, and can produce varices secondary to portal obstruction with a potential risk of haemorrhage.

e. True The middle 1 cm zone shows the greatest rise in pressure on manometry.

54. *Synopsis 397; Scott-Brown 1/10/31–32, 1/11/7–9, 5/24/2*

a. False There is no thickening of the circular muscle layer, and this is therefore called a 'physiological' sphincter.

b. False It is produced by the right crus, as it splits to encircle the oesophagus.

c. True The folds may have a valvular effect.

d. False Acid reflux can occur despite a normal angle. However, the sharp angle may act as a mechanical flap valve.

e. False The sling is the oblique muscle fibres of the stomach encircling the lower oesophagus. However, this site does not correspond to the sphincteric mechanism, and the anti-reflux mechanism is still present after section of the sling fibres.

55. **Congenital atresia of the oesophagus:**
    a. Most cases of oesophageal atresia are associated with a tracheo-oesophageal fistula.
    b. Gas in the gastro-intestinal tract implies the presence of polyhydramnios.
    c. Feeding is likely to produce aspiration pneumonitis.
    d. After successful surgical correction, swallowing develops normally.
    e. Mortality is primarily related to the site of the defect.

56. **Hiatus hernia:**
    a. A para-oesophageal hernia is more likely to produce reflux than a sliding hernia.
    b. Dysphagia is the most common presenting complaint.
    c. A gastric air shadow is seen in the sliding variety.
    d. Surgery is particularly indicated in para-oesophageal herniae.
    e. Nissen fundoplication is contraindicated in children.

55. *Synopsis 398–400; Scott-Brown 6/29/1–7*
   a. True   The majority will be distal fistulae. In the neonate, these can lead to aspiration of meconium.
   b. False   Gas in the gastro-intestinal tract below the atresia indicates the presence of a tracheo-oesophageal fistula. Polyhydramnios occurs in 30 per cent of mothers, due to the inability of the foetus to swallow amniotic fluid.
   c. True   This is caused either by overspill into the trachea, or via a tracheo-oesophageal fistula. If atresia is suspected, the first feed should be withheld.
   d. False   Difficulties may persist for years due to stricture or oesophageal dysmobility.
   e. False   This is dependent on associated abnormalities, particularly cardiac defects.

56. *Synopsis 401, 414; Scott-Brown 5/24/12–13, 6/29/13–18*
   a. False   The reverse is true. In the para-oesophageal hernia, the gastro-oesophageal function is retained below the diaphragm but a portion of the stomach protrudes through the hiatus. Mixed herniae can occur.
   b. False   The commonest symptoms are heartburn and retrosternal discomfort.
   c. False   This is seen in the para-oesophageal type on a lateral chest X-ray, and is located posterior to the heart.
   d. True   This is to prevent complications such as anaemia and pseudo-angina (obstruction or impaction).
   e. False   This is the mainstay of surgical treatment, both in children and adults.

57. **Perforation of the oesophagus:**
    a. Perforation is more likely to occur with a flexible than with a rigid oesophagoscope.
    b. Severe vomiting may produce a tear in the middle third of the oesophagus.
    c. Severe back or chest pain with cervical surgical emphysema is pathognomonic.
    d. If treatment is delayed more than 24 hours, the mortality is about 50 per cent.
    e. Contrast radiology should not be performed because of the risk of chemical mediastinitis.

58. **Clinical features of a foreign body in the oesophagus include the following:**
    a. Back pain.
    b. Hoarseness.
    c. Dyspnoea.
    d. The absence of laryngeal crepitus.
    e. Excessive salivation.

57. *Synopsis 402–404; Scott-Brown 5/1/3,8–9, 5/24/5, 20–21*
a. False   Rigid oesophagoscopy has the higher perforation rate, but is used in a different group of patients. For example, the rigid endoscope is necessary for the removal of large, sharp foreign bodies. These cases carry a much higher risk of perforation than the routine flexible oesophagogastroduodenoscopy for dyspepsia.
b. False   These tears most frequently occur in the lower end as a longitudinal tear involving all layers of the viscus.
c. True   However, if the thoracic oesophagus is involved, surgical emphysema may be absent. Air under the diaphragm may be present in ruptures of the abdominal portion.
d. True   Early diagnosed cervical tears may be managed conservatively, but thoracic tears rarely respond to medical treatment. Surgery for repair and/or drainage should not be delayed if the clinical picture demands it.
e. False   This will delineate the site and aetiology of perforation. Dionysil opaque medium should be used.

58. *Synopsis 404–406; Scott-Brown 5/1/11–12, 5/24/21–22, 6/29/10–12*
a. True   Pain is referred to the back or retrosternum, particularly if the foreign object is in the middle or lower third of the oesophagus and therefore poorly localized.
b. True   Impaction at the cricopharyngeal sphincter may lead to laryngeal oedema.
c. True   This is for the same reason as (b) and, in children, because the trachea may be compressed by the foreign object.
d. True   This is due to oesophageal oedema. Localized tenderness is present on laryngeal palpation.
e. True   This occurs because saliva pools in the pyriform fossae.

59. Benign neoplasms of the oesophagus:
a. These account for about 25 per cent of oesophageal neoplasms.
b. Smooth muscle tumours are the most common.
c. They may be regurgitated into the mouth.
d. Leiomyomas are readily visualized during endoscopy.
e. Dysphagia is uncommon.

60. Carcinoma of the oesophagus:
a. Environmental factors account for large regional variations in incidence.
b. This tends to develop at the sites of normal narrowing.
c. Achalasia is a risk factor.
d. Cigarette smoking is not a risk factor.
e. Carcinoma of the oesophagus is more common in females than in males.

59. *Synopsis 407; Scott-Brown 5/24/23*
a. False Less than 10 per cent of oesophageal neoplasms are benign.
b. True These account for about 60 per cent of all benign tumours.
c. True This is particularly so if they are pedunculated and located in the upper oesophagus.
d. False They are submucosal and are easily missed. A barium swallow will show a characteristic smooth filling defect.
e. True The main symptom is the feeling of a lump in the throat, only latterly producing dysphagia.

60. *Synopsis 407–410; Scott-Brown 5/24/16–20*
a. True Factors vary. They include ingestion of nitrosamine carcinogens from cooking pots by Bantu tribesmen, and excessive consumption of home-distilled Calvados in Normandy.
b. True Carcinoma of the oesophagus tends to develop particularly at the junction of the pharynx and oesophagus, and where the aorta and left main bronchus cross.
c. True The prevalence is 3–7 per cent in achalasics, and the disease occurs at a younger age.
d. False Cigarette smoking is a risk factor, and the risk multiplies with high alcohol consumption.
e. False Over 75 per cent of patients are male.

61. Management of oesophageal cancer:
√ a.   The right colon is the most suitable portion of the colon for interposition.
√ b.   The argon laser is a useful tool for the vaporization of tumour.
  c.   The Mousseau-Barbin tube is designed to be pushed through a tumour stricture, over an endoscopically placed guide wire.
  d.   Radiotherapy is likely to produce radiation corditis.
√ e.   Gastrostomy is essential to maintain nutrition after resection.

62. Oesophageal stricture:
√ a.   This is most commonly due to reflux oesophagitis.
  b.   Endoscopy is not required if barium studies reveal a smooth narrowing.
  c.   The Shatskis ring can cause narrowing.
  d.   Stricture may be caused by ingesting potassium salts.
  e.   Peptic reflux strictures should be bouginaged if causing dysphagia.

√√ **63. Achalasia of the cardia:**
√ a.   There is abnormal peristalsis in the lower oesophagus.
  b.   Meissner's ganglion cells in the oesophagus are absent.
  c.   Amyl nitrate inhalation is the treatment of choice.
  d.   Ramstedt's operation relieves symptoms in the majority of patients.
  e.   Oesophagectasia is present.

61. *Synopsis 407–410; Scott-Brown 5/24/18–20*
  a. False The right side is bulky, and it has a tenuous blood supply at the ileo-caecal region. The left colon is preferred due to its lesser bulk, comparable calibre and ability to propel solid material. Microvascular free jejunal grafts may be employed for high resections.
  b. False The neodymium YAG laser is employed, as it passes down a flexible tube. It is particularly useful for recurrences at anastomotic sites and high lesions.
  c. False It was designed to be pulled through the tumour via a gastrostomy. However, it can be placed endoscopically over a guide wire following Eder-Puestow dilatation.
  d. False Radiation pneumonitis and post-radiation stricture may occur. Radiotherapy is usually palliative if surgery is not contemplated.
  e. False Nasogastric or parenteral feeding allows the anastomosis time to heal. Gastrostomy as a form of palliation is not justified.

62. *Synopsis 410–411; Scott-Brown 5/1/6, 5/2/14–16, 5/24/11–13, 6/29/13–18*
  a. True.
  b. False Endoscopy should be carried out in all cases, to exclude a neoplasm and to assess the precise level and severity of the lesion.
  c. True This is a lower oesophageal web similar to the cervical web at the pharyngo-oesophageal junction (Paterson-Brown-Kelly or Plummer-Vinson syndrome).
  d. True Potassium in diuretic preparations may cause oesophagitis, with subsequent narrowing.
  e. True This should be combined with intensive medical treatment to neutralize acid.

63. *Synopsis 411–413; Scott-Brown 5/2/17, 5/24/11–12, 6/29/7–10*
  a. False Peristalsis is absent.
  b. False There is an absence or reduction in cells in Auerbach's plexus.
  c. False This may be improve swallowing before meals, but surgical treatment is favoured.
  d. False Ramstedt's operation is a myotomy for infantile pyloric stenosis. Heller's operation, which is also a myotomy, is employed in achalasia, with excellent symptomatic relief.
  e. True Achalasia and oesophagectasia are synonyms.

General and related topics

1. **Principles of radiotherapy:**
   a. Cobalt-60 produces gamma radiation.
   b. Megavoltage beams from linear accelerators produce marked skin reactions.
   c. Bone necrosis is more likely if the total dose delivered is by orthovoltage beams.
   d. Electron absorption is directly proportional to their energy level.
   e. X-rays are a form of piezo-electric radiation.

2. **Efficacy of radiotherapy:**
   a. Squamous cell tumours are more responsive than tumours of lymphoid origin.
   b. Sarcomata of bony origin have a very poor response rate.
   √ c. The efficacy of radiotherapy is enhanced by hypothermia.
   d. Photons damage cells more effectively than neutrons.
   e. Hypoxia protects tumour cells.

1. *Synopsis – no specific reference; Scott-Brown 1/21/1–10*
   a. True   A disadvantage of Cobalt-60 is that it decays and has to be replaced every 3–5 years.
   b. False   They are skin-sparing, as the maximum dose is delivered deep to the skin. Orthovoltage beams are useful for superficial skin tumours.
   c. True   This is because bone has low transmission and high absorption rates. However, megavoltage beams allow satisfactory tissue absorption and minimize bone absorption.
   d. True   Electrons have a finite absorption depth, and are therefore useful in treating superficial lesions or a block of tissue of known dimensions.
   e. False   X-rays are a type of electromagnetic radiation.

2. *Synopsis – no specific reference; Scott-Brown 1/21/1–10*
   a. False   The reverse is true. Anaplastic and embryonal tumours also have a high response rate, but recurrence rates are significant.
   b. True.
   c. False   Hyperthermia enhances the response to radiotherapy, but it is difficult to achieve a temperature difference between tumour and surrounding normal tissue.
   d. False   Neutrons are more destructive, as they are highly charged and densely ionizing. However, the therapeutic ratio is almost one, and hence normal tissue is frequently damaged.
   e. True   This explains the use of hyperbaric oxygen chambers to enhance the effect of radiotherapy. However, normal tissue also becomes more richly oxygenated, with increased risk of necrosis, and there are great practical difficulties with access to the patient in pressurization tanks. Barotrauma is also a problem; some patients require grommets.

√ 3. **During a course of radical radiotherapy for head and neck cancer:**
   a. Endarteritis in blood vessels may induce bony necrosis of the maxilla.
   √ b. Radiation mucositis is a sign that the limit of tissue tolerance has been reached.
   c. The commonest infection in the oral cavity is *Aspergillus fumigatus*.
   d. Wet shaving is essential to remove the hair growth that impairs therapy.
   e. A rest period is essential every 5 days.

4. **Cytotoxic agents in head and neck cancer:**
   a. Cell destruction follows first-order kinetics.
   b. Cycle-specific drugs destroy both resting and cycling cells equally.
   c. Methotrexate is a phase-specific agent.
   d. Synchronization means all the cells passing in phase through the cell cycle.
   e. Folic acid acts by enhancing the therapeutic effect of methotrexate.

5. **Adjuvant chemotherapy in head and neck cancer:**
   a. Impaired renal function precludes the use of methotrexate.
   b. A combination of class III anti-tumour drugs can be given in normal doses.
   c. Pulmonary fibrosis develops in 10 per cent of patients on bleomycin.
   d. Cisplatin has a cumulative toxic side effect.
   e. The term 'no response' indicates a reduction of between 50 and 70 per cent in the product of the two largest perpendicular diameters of measurable tumour.

3. *Synopsis – no specific reference; Scott-Brown 1/21/1–10*
a. True However, this is a particular problem in the mandible.
b. True Trauma, alcohol, tobacco should be avoided, as these enhance the problem. Pain is an associated feature.
c. False *Candida albicans* is the most common infection. Treatment is by continuous local antifungal therapy in the form of nystatin lozenges, or other appropriate preparation.
d. False An electric razor should be employed to avoid excessive trauma to the skin.
e. False Conventionally, radiotherapy is given during weekdays; the 'rest period' is really for the staff at weekends. There is some evidence that these rest periods should be avoided, as the tumour has a chance to recover. Hyper-fractionation techniques typically involve giving the treatment three times daily for 12 days without a break.

4. *Synopsis – no specific reference; Scott-Brown 1/22/1–20*
a. True A given drug dose kills a constant fraction of cells, regardless of the total number of tumour cells present.
b. False The latter are more sensitive. Cyclophosphamide is an example.
c. True It destroys proliferating cells during a specific part of the cell cycle.
d. True.
e. False It reverses the toxic side effects, and is employed as 'rescue' therapy for the bone marrow after giving a deliberate overdose of methotrexate. Unfortunately, the tumour may also be rescued.

5. *Synopsis – no specific reference; Scott-Brown 1/22/1–20*
a. False The folinic acid rescue can be extended in such cases.
b. False Class III combinations should be given in proportionately reduced doses, as normal bone marrow stem cells are killed by increasing dosages.
c. False Pulmonary fibrosis develops in only about 1 per cent of these patients. However, 10 per cent develop a non-specific pneumonitis.
d. True These side effects are reduced by adequate prehydration and by maintaining a diuresis. Major side effects include nephrotoxicity, ototoxicity and haematological effects.
e. False This term indicates either no change in size, or less than a 50 per cent reduction of measurable tumour.

6. **Principles of surgical lasers:**
   a. A laser beam is collimated.
   b. The thermal effects include contraction of collagen.
   c. Vaporization is produced by boiling of intracellular water.
   d. Interaction of a Nd-YAG laser with tissue produces zones of vaporization and coagulation.
   e. At low power, surgical lasers may produce biostimulation.

7. **The carbon dioxide laser:**
   a. Light is absorbed by water.
   b. This can seal blood vessels up to 1.5 mm in diameter.
   c. Nerve endings are sealed.
   d. Skin incisions heal with greater rapidity than conventional scalpel wounds.
   e. The light beam can be transmitted by flexible fibres.

6. *Synopsis – no specific reference; Scott-Brown 1/25/1–10*
   a. True   That is, parallel. It is also monochromatic, of a single
             wavelength and in phase.
   b. True   If the tissue temperature rises above 60°C, protein is
             denatured and this produces contraction. This effect
             accounts for the haemostatic properties of laser light.
   c. True.
   d. True   It also produces a zone of cell death, which is replaced
             by fibrous tissue without loss of physical integrity. This
             makes the Nd-YAG laser particularly useful for
             palliation of tumours in the oesophagus, as there is
             little risk of perforation.
   e. True   This can enhance wound healing.

7. *Synopsis – no specific reference; Scott-Brown 1/25/7–8*
   a. True   Since most soft tissues comprise between 75 and 90 per
              cent water, light absorption induces boiling and a rapid
              increase in volume.
   b. False   It can seal blood vessels only up to 0.5 mm in diameter.
              By defocusing the beam slightly, larger vessels can be
              sealed. The argon laser is more effective in coagulating
              blood vessels; hence its use in ophthalmological
              vascular pathologies.
   c. True   This may account for the reduction in pain after CO_2
              laser surgery. Lymphatics are also sealed, and this may
              reduce the risk of spread of malignant cells.
   d. False   Skin incisions heal more slowly and initially are of
              poorer tensile strength.
   e. False   This is not the case for the CO_2 laser. The Nd-YAG
              and KTP beams can be transmitted by fibreoptic cable.

✓ 8. **The safe use of lasers:**
   a. A room in which a medical laser is operated must have an illuminated warning sign and a klaxon, and the doors must be automatically locked to visitors when the device is active.
   b. Metal plating of flexible anaesthetic tubes prevents the possibility of ignition.
   c. Plain glass spectacles will protect the eye from CO_2 laser light.
   d. A laser safety officer is responsible for maintaining a list of nominated users.
   e. Protective clothing is essential to avoid skin injury.

✓✓ 9. **Clinical applications of lasers in otolaryngology:**
   ✓ a. The CO_2 laser produces a greater remission rate than interferon in cases of recurrent respiratory papillomatosis.
   b. A Nd-YAG laser is particularly useful for the removal of intubation granuloma from the vocal cords.
   c. The KTP and argon lasers can be applied via a flexible fibreoptic cable to vaporize the crura in small fenestra stapedotomy.
   d. The CO_2 laser can be used to provide precise dermabrasion in treatment of rhinophyma.
   e. Division of thick vocal cord webs is very successful.

8. *Synopsis – no specific reference; Scott-Brown 1/25/11–15*
   a. False Warning signs must be posted but not necessarily
   illuminated. A klaxon is not required. Although access
   should be limited to those personnel essential to the
   procedure, current regulations do not specify
   automatic locking of the doors to visitors.
   b. False Ignition may still occur if tubes are surrounded by
   oxygen and nitrous oxide. The metal coating may not
   completely cover the plastic, and cracks can appear in it.
   c. False The spectacles have to attenuate the laser beam to
   below the maximum permissible exposure. The
   patient's eyes can be protected with pads soaked in
   water, eye shields or steel contact lenses.
   d. True This is usually a medical physicist.
   e. False Unless a direct beam strikes the skin, the damage is
   insignificant.

9. *Synopsis – no specific reference; Scott-Brown 1/25/15–21*
   a. False Interferon produces excellent regression, but with
   rapid recurrence when treatment is withdrawn.
   b. False The Nd-YAG is too blunt an instrument for this
   procedure, and causes deep tissue burns which would
   be deleterious on the vocal cords. The CO_2 laser is
   ideally suited for this treatment because it is precise
   and does not penetrate deeply.
   c. True Laser crurotomy is particularly indicated in small
   fenestra techniques. It reduces the risk of footplate
   fracture or avulsion.
   d. True.
   e. False These are usually post-traumatic lesions, and the
   recurrence rate is high. Keels are required to prevent
   recurrence.

✓✓ **10. Photodynamic therapy:**
    a. The phthalocyanines are the most widely used tumour sensitizers.
    b. Destruction of tissue is by the cytotoxic effect of triplet oxygen.
  ✓ c. Skin photosensitization lasts up to 7 days.
    d. Haematoporphyrin derivative (HPD) is activated at 630 mm and is wavelength selective.
    e. Retention of sensitizer is related to its ingestion by malignant cells.

✓✓ **11. Local anaesthetic and vasoconstrictor agents used in ENT**
    a. In the early stages of cocaine toxicity, there is a rise in blood pressure and respiratory rate.
  ✓ b. The maximum dose of adrenaline by injection is 0.5 mg in a fit adult.
    c. A low pH in tissue will render local anaesthesia less effective.
    d. Felypressin has a greater effect on the myocardium than adrenaline.
    e. If adrenaline is contraindicated, prilocaine may be employed.

12. Biomaterials in otolaryngology:
    a. A biotolerant material does not produce a foreign body reaction.
    b. Plastipore and proplast are porous alloplasts, which allow ingrowth of fibrous tissue and capillaries.
    c. Ceravital is a bioactive glass ceramic.
    d. Calcium phosphate ceramics have high tensile strength.
    e. Cobalt–chromium alloys are corrosion resistant.

10. *Synopsis – no specific reference; Scott-Brown 1/25/2–3, 21*
  a. False Haematoporphyrin derivative is the most widely used tumour sensitizer. However, the tumour to normal tissue take-up ratio is low. Experimentally the phthalocyanines have a much higher ratio, and these may prove to be ideal sensitizers.
  b. False Cytotoxic singlet oxygen is produced after activation of HPD.
  c. False Skin photosensitization lasts 6–8 weeks.
  d. True This allows a depth of penetration of 1 cm. HPD is best activated by UV light, but the depth of penetration is poor.
  e. False The abnormal tumour circulation retains the sensitizer. The cells do not take up tumour sensitizer.

11. *Synopsis – no specific reference; Scott-Brown 1/27/5–10*
  a. True This may be dramatic if hypersensitivity is present. Later, the blood pressure may crash, with ventricular fibrillation, convulsions and respiratory arrest.
  b. True That is about 100 ml of the standard 1:200 000 solution, or 0.5 ml of the 1:1000 solution.
  c. True Acid pH (e.g. in pus and inflamed tissue) increases the ionized particles in the drug and inactivates it.
  d. False It has much lower systemic effects; however, it takes longer to produce vasoconstrictor effects.
  e. True Prilocaine is less toxic. High doses may produce cyanosis due to methaemoglobin formation.

12. *Synopsis – no specific reference; Scott-Brown 1/28/1–7*
  a. False There is an initial reaction, which ceases after incorporation.
  b. True These gained popularity in middle ear reconstruction, but the extrusion rate is high.
  c. True This allows bonding between the implant and living tissue. Some degradation takes place. It can be difficult to shape when employed in the middle ear.
  d. False They are very brittle. Hydroxyapatite and B Whitlockite have been employed in otology. The former is more biodegradable, and may not be replaced by new bone as quickly as it disappears.
  e. True They are used in mandibular reconstruction.

13. **Medical negligence in otolaryngology:**
    a. Medical negligence is proved if there has been a breach of duty of care by the doctor.
    b. The Bolam test in English law establishes that the doctor is not negligent if acting in accordance with a practice supported by a reasonable body of medical opinion, even if this is a minority view.
    c. 'Informed consent' in English law means that all conceivable risks must be listed.
    d. Damage to the facial nerve during mastoid surgery for cholesteatoma is negligent.
    e. Perforation of the oesophagus during removal of a foreign body is negligent.

13. *Synopsis – no specific reference; Scott-Brown 1/29/1–13*

a. False   Proof of negligence requires in addition that the breach of duty of care has caused damage to the plaintiff. Even if it is clear that the doctor failed in the duty of care and behaved in a negligent way, the case will fail unless the plaintiff can go on to show that the injury is directly attributable to the doctor's poor performance.

b. True   This allows for the inevitable diversity of view within the specialty. The Bolam case also established that a practitioner does not have to possess the highest expert skill, only that of the ordinary skilled doctor within that specialty.

c. False   Only common or serious risks need be mentioned at present.

d. False   This is not necessarily negligent, as the nerve may be dehiscent or aberrant. However, failure to warn of the possibility beforehand and failure to recognize and manage the complication at the time would, taken together with the nerve injury, make a case difficult to defend.

e. False   This is not necessarily negligent, as the foreign body itself may cause the perforation. Rigid oesophagoscopy should be carried out by adequately trained staff, and trainees must be closely supervised until competent. Failure to recognize and treat the perforation at an early stage would probably constitute negligence.